HOLISTIC HYPNOBIRTHING

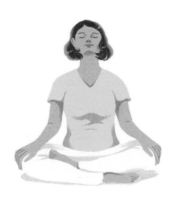

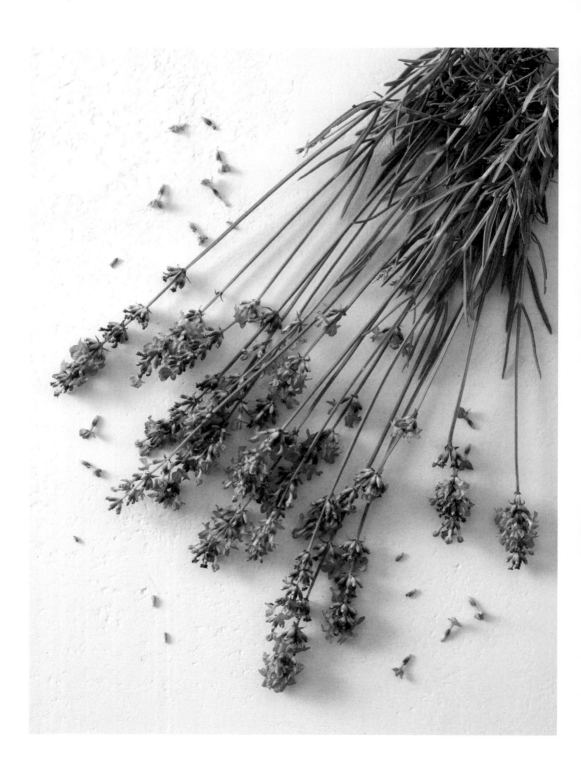

HOLISTIC HYPNOBIRTHING

Mindful Practices for a Positive
Pregnancy and Birth

Anthonissa Moger

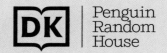

Senior Editor Salima Hirani
Project Designer Vanessa Hamilton
Senior Designer Barbara Zuniga
US Editor Jennette ElNaggar
Editorial Assistant Kiron Gill
Jacket Designer Amy Cox
Senior Production Editor Tony Phipps
Senior Producer Luca Bazzoli
Creative Technical Support Sonia Charbonnier
Managing Editor Dawn Henderson
Managing Art Editor Marianne Markham
Art Director Maxine Pedliham
Publishing Director Katie Cowan

Illustrator Mikyung Lee
Photographer Ruth Jenkinson
Food Stylist Tamara Vos
Prop Stylist Robert Merrett

First American Edition, 2021
Published in the United States by DK Publishing
1450 Broadway, Suite 801, New York, NY 10018

Published in Great Britain by Dorling Kindersley Limited.

A catalog record for this book is available
from the Library of Congress.
ISBN 978-0-7440-2685-6

Printed and bound in China

For the curious

www.dk.com

MIX
Paper from
responsible sources
FSC™ C018179

This book was made with Forest Stewardship Council™
certified paper—one small step in DK's commitment to
a sustainable future. For more information go to
www.dk.com/our-green-pledge

Contents

foreword

Our bodies innately know how to birth our babies. You have within you all the strength, resilience, and peace you need to enjoy a truly empowering and positive birth experience. Hypnobirthing can help you tap into these infinite natural resources.

Growing up, I inherited powerful birth stories from my mother, who said she could have birthed in nature without assistance. This instilled a strong belief in myself and my birthing body. I approached my first birth with a few good books and no fear. I was lucky enough to see the same midwife throughout my pregnancy, and she happened to be on call when I went into labor. She was calm, quiet, respectful, and made me feel safe. My daughter Jazz was born at home in 2008. The intense, enjoyable experience catapulted me into motherhood feeling healthy, passionate, and inspired, and it soon became clear that midwifery was my calling. I began my training when Jazz turned one. My interest in natural birthing meant that hypnobirthing became part of the picture.

As an NHS midwife, I have attended many home births and now work on a busy labor ward in central London. I see firsthand the difference between women who prepare their minds and bodies for birth using hypnobirthing tools and those who come in unprepared, anxious, and afraid. The former are more calm, confident, comfortable during the birth and better able to navigate special circumstances, if they arise.

When you harness the power of your mind, believe in your body, learn how to relax deeply, and choose to give birth in a comfortable environment, supported by a caring team, you inevitably change your birthing experience for the better.

"

Give birth with confidence, in a powerful state of euphoria.

"

We are animals with an instinctive ability to give birth, and practices developed over millennia to help us do so. We are also modern humans with advanced medical care at our disposal. As a hypnobirthing midwife, I feel privileged to bridge the gap between the two worlds.

In this book, trimester by trimester I'll show you how to use hypnobirthing techniques, complementary therapies, and natural remedies to give birth to your baby as nature intended yet in a modern context (whether that's a hospital or your own home), with the help of a midwife who, like me, is working from the basis of their scientific training. I share the best of what I have learned over a decade as a midwife and an instructor of yoga and hypnobirthing. I have practiced everything within these pages myself—I wrote this book while pregnant with my son Indy. Writing each trimester as I experienced it has shaped the book, and I have included only the most practical and beneficial content.

I hope you will find this guidance helpful, and I wish you a wonderful journey into motherhood. Remember—you are designed to do this!

Anthonissa

INTRODUCTION

what is hypnobirthing?

Hypnobirthing is a practical philosophy that incorporates
a range of tools and techniques designed to help you
prepare your body and mind for birth during pregnancy
and experience giving birth as a joyful life event.

Although hypnobirthing has become increasingly popular in recent years, it is nothing new. Women have been birthing using the breath, supported by family and community midwives, in a cozy, safe environment since time immemorial. It is only in recent times that we have come to recognize and appreciate how beneficial these factors are for having a straightforward and positive experience.

HYPNOBIRTHING PHILOSOPHY
At the heart of hypnobirthing is the belief that the body has a built-in capacity to give birth. Understanding this ability in your own body (see pp.106–107) and learning how to work with (not against) it, using breathing techniques and deep relaxation through self-hypnosis (see pp.16–17), can help you birth your baby in a way that is closer to how nature intended.

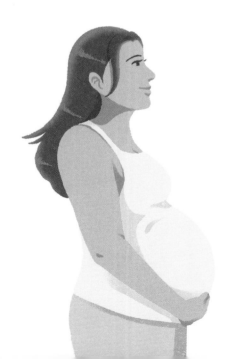

"

Hypnobirthing promotes a healthy, peaceful pregnancy and birth, benefitting mom and baby.

"

It is commonly believed that childbirth is an unavoidably painful or traumatic experience, something to be approached with fear and endured by women. This is not the case. Hypnobirthing retrains your state of mind and emotions to reframe birth as one of life's most fulfilling seminal moments, an event that can be celebrated and enjoyed, in a calm environment created by yourself, in which you feel safe and nurtured.

HYPNOBIRTHING IN PRACTICE

There are four aspects to hypnobirthing practice: relaxation, mindset work, body preparation, and teamwork. Prepare your body for birth with gentle, targeted exercise. At the same time, learn relaxation skills and nurture your mental and emotional state using mindset tools so you approach the birth feeling strong, confident, and relaxed.

Surround yourself with a coterie of supporters—your partner and/or birth partner, the medical professionals involved, and anyone who makes you feel nurtured and safe. Practice using your hypnobirthing tools with their help as much as possible.

With such preparation, hypnobirthing moms experience birth as a joyous event, and happy moms make for happy babies.

designed to give birth

Hypnobirthing celebrates women's bodies as capable, powerful, and designed to birth. It encourages and teaches women to work with their innate birthing ability to birth their babies in a state similar to how other mammals give birth in nature.

We give birth within the context of a medicalized approach, so it's easy to forget that female bodies are designed for birth. Although medical professionals and procedures are there to support us, by using hypnobirthing techniques, you optimize your chance of a straightforward birth and reduce the likelihood of needing medical interventions.

Women's incredible bodies have evolved to birth our babies in amazing ways. The purpose of the uterus is to nurture the growth of a baby and, when the right time comes, uterine muscles can exert powerful pressure from the top and sides, squeezing the baby down and opening the cervix (see p.107).

We have a wide pelvis compared to men, enabling a baby to pass through it. The hormone relaxin also peaks around birth, relaxing the pelvic ligaments so this capacity can increase further, and the coccyx (tailbone) becomes more flexible to enable it to move 1–2cm to allow the baby through.

BIRTHING HORMONES
The two main types of hormone the body uses during childbirth are oxytocin and endorphins.

"
Allow your body's wisdom
to be your guide.
"

Oxytocin is known as the hormone of love. It makes us feel safe and relaxed. We release an abundance of it at many times throughout our lives, including when we fall in love, receive a massage, hold hands or cuddle, have an orgasm, eat delicious food, and when we give birth to, and breastfeed, our babies. During birth, oxytocin causes the surges that open the cervix and bring the baby down, so the more of it you have flowing, the more likely it is that your birth will be comparatively short and comfortable. Oxytocin levels in the body rise significantly throughout pregnancy, and the uterus itself develops oxytocin receptors in order to prime it for birthing.

Endorphins are morphine the body makes itself. With the right conditions (being calm and relaxed), your body will release this potent natural painkiller into your system abundantly, which is extremely helpful during birth.

Using hypnobirthing techniques, you learn to tune in to your body to support the production of birthing hormones as you tap in to the innate birthing wisdom of your body, just as any other mammal does when the time comes to give birth.

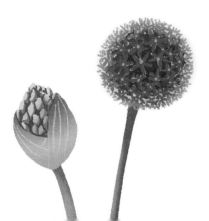

INTRODUCTION

mind-body connection

The mind and body are one, working together symbiotically,
so when we believe in ourselves, the body responds on
a physiological level. This means a positive
mindset can be life-changing.

Thoughts affect the body on every level—including the hormones that regulate all body systems. Your perceptions of the world inform your nervous system, which responds accordingly.

The autonomic nervous system is part of the central nervous system and is responsible for the body's unconscious functions. It has two divisions: the sympathetic nervous system and the parasympathetic nervous system.

If under stress, the sympathetic nervous system kicks into action, mobilizing the famous fight-or-flight response that enables your body to respond to a perceived threat. Your system is flooded with the hormones adrenaline and cortisol, allowing you to respond quickly to danger. Breathing and heart rates increase, muscles tense in order to fight or take flight, and nonessential body systems shut down to divert all resources to survival.

THE KEY TO CALMNESS
The parasympathetic nervous system is the counterbalance to the sympathetic nervous system. It is activated if you perceive a threat has passed or whenever you are calm. It lowers your heart rate and blood pressure, reduces levels of the stress hormones adrenaline and cortisol, relaxes the muscles, returns breathing to a steady state, and activates body systems not involved in urgent self-defense. For

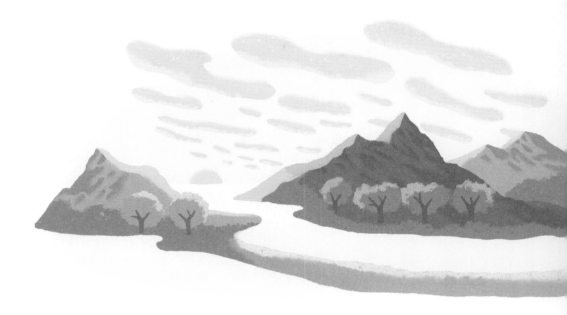

instance, the parasympathetic nervous system improves immunity and enables cellular healing.

During childbirth, intense fear and stress tend to slow down, delay, or even switch off the birthing process, as your body perceives a threat and delays birthing until it has passed. The presence of the stress hormones cortisol and adrenaline suppresses the release of the birthing hormone oxytocin as well as endorphins, the body's natural painkillers (see p.11). If you are calm, the natural birthing process remains uninhibited.

Only one division of the autonomic nervous system can be active at any time. This means the single most important thing you can do to promote a smooth birth is to soothe your stress response and remain as calm as possible, to keep the parasympathetic system activated. Hypnobirthing helps you do this through tools that enable deep relaxation and by harnessing the power of the mind.

INTRODUCTION

harnessing the mind

Because the mind exerts a strong influence on the body, by harnessing its power you work with your body to give birth with increased ease. Use the hypnobirthing tools in this book throughout pregnancy to nurture a positive mindset about birthing.

A positive approach to childbirth can become a self-fulfilling prophecy. Moms who are calm and confident have boosted levels of oxytocin and endorphins (see p.11), leading to a smoother, quicker, more comfortable labor and birth. If special circumstances occur, those moms who can remain calm are in a good state of mind to make the right choices for themselves in the moment and come out of the experience feeling empowered. A positive mindset helps them accept the unplanned outcome while remaining connected to the magic of the event.

Not everyone finds it easy to be positive, especially when facing the unknown or after a previous difficult birth. The good news is that your mind is flexible due to neuroplasticity. With a little hypnobirthing practice, you can change the pathways and synapses in your brain, deleting those that no longer serve you (negative thoughts) and strengthening those that support a positive approach to giving birth.

MINDSET TOOLS

The tools in this book can help you develop positive thinking habits. They

"

Work on developing a positive mindset—
this is where your power lies.

"

enable you to take control of your mind and emotions through nurturing them, to build mental and emotional resilience, strength, and confidence. Don't feel you have to do all the exercises—use only those that resonate with you. Use them to help you reframe individual negative thoughts as positive ones. This is an ongoing process, done gradually over days and weeks. Each time you have a negative thought about pregnancy or birth, or life beyond birth, replace it with a positive one, so you build confidence one positive thought at a time.

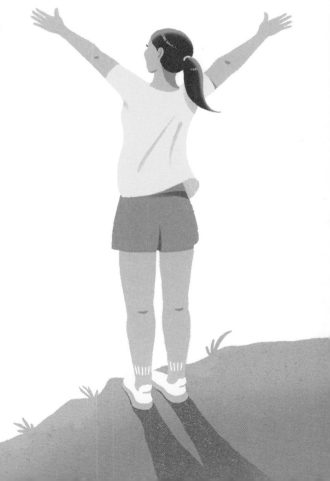

INTRODUCTION

self-hypnosis

During pregnancy and childbirth, hypnobirthing moms use self-hypnosis techniques to enter a deep state of relaxation. In this pleasurable state of consciousness, limiting and negative beliefs can be released from the subconscious mind.

Hypnobirthing gets its name from the self-hypnosis involved. Some people worry about the idea of hypnosis. Be reassured that it does not mean that you will be in a trance and unaware of your surroundings. Rather, you will be aware of everything that is going on around you yet in a deeply relaxed state and hyper-tuned in to your own birthing body.

You can use self-hypnosis tools such as visualization and breathing techniques to invoke a deep state of relaxation. Brain waves slow down as you enter the theta brain state, during which the subconscious mind becomes accessible and you can implant into it your chosen beliefs.

Women who are calm and relaxed during birth enter a hypnotic state naturally due to their high levels of

"

Tap in to your subconscious mind to release anxiety and increase confidence.

"

oxytocin and endorphins (see p.13). Self-hypnosis during birth allows you to tune in to your body, boost these hormones, and work with the birthing process to promote a comfortable experience. Your perception of time shrinks when in this state—an hour can feel like 5 minutes—so the birth seems shorter. Try the self-hypnosis tools in this book and practice those that appeal to you.

INTRODUCTION

your tool kit

Use the exercises in this book to help you build your holistic hypnobirthing tool kit trimester by trimester to prepare for the birth. Follow your instincts when selecting from the various tools, focusing on those that feel good.

BREATH WORK

The breath is a powerful hypnobirthing tool. Slow breathing activates the parasympathetic nervous system (see p.12), increasing feelings of calm and promoting the presence of birthing hormones (see p.10). I have included several useful breathing exercises, and in Chapter 4, you'll find techniques specially designed for the different stages of birth. Practice these techniques regularly throughout pregnancy to teach yourself to drop down into a state of deep relaxation within 1–2 minutes.

RELAXATION AND VISUALIZATION

Self-hypnosis techniques help you enter a state of deep relaxation. The exercises in this book are easy to follow. If you find it difficult to remember the steps, have your partner/birth partner read them out to you when you practice. Alternatively, record yourself reading out the steps and allow your own voice to guide you through the exercise. When it comes to visualization, don't be disheartened if you find it difficult to conjure mental pictures—not everyone can. Just focus on how the exercise makes you feel.

MINDSET DEVELOPMENT

The mindset exercises in this book help you tune in to yourself with compassion, release unhelpful thoughts, and foster confidence. They are not meant to be a chore but something that feels nurturing and nourishing, so pick those that appeal to you. It might feel hard to dig in to your psyche and grapple with difficult emotions, but facing things that worry you is the best way to feel less worried. With a little practice, it becomes easier.

"

A holistic approach prepares both body and mind for this wonderful adventure.

"

BODY WORK

Learn to tune in to your body and its changing needs during each trimester. Use the guidance in this book to strengthen and tone your body, ease aches and pains, and encourage your baby into a good position for birth. You'll find yoga sequences tailored for different stages of pregnancy, and I encourage you to walk, swim, and practice other forms of mindful movement as well as use natural remedies and alternative therapies to nurture body and mind. Many women report that aromatherapy, acupuncture, reflexology, reiki, and osteopathy help ease common ailments and lift the mood.

Massage is also important in the hypnobirthing tool kit. Physical touch boosts useful hormones, relieves backache, and promotes connection

with your partner. On pp.122–125, you'll find massage techniques that have helped many women during birth. Ask your partner or birth partner to practice these on you during pregnancy so you learn together how to make them work for you.

TEAMWORK

Build your team during pregnancy so you feel supported. During the next few months, you will begin to identify the people in your life who make the pregnancy feel like a positive and empowering experience. Draw those people in closer so you have emotional and practical support from a reliable team. If you have a partner, the partner exercises in this book will help you connect as parents of your growing baby and work as a team during pregnancy, birth, and beyond.

INTRODUCTION

positive language

Words have a profound effect on the psyche. Positive language
helps create a positive mindset and, conversely, negative language,
a negative one. Hypnobirthing employs the power of language to
help you feel empowered about giving birth.

AFFIRMATIONS

Setting intentions for how you want to think, feel, and act can lead to tangible results, as your focus guides your thoughts and actions. Affirmations can support this process.

An affirmation is a short statement used to direct your focus and promote positive thinking. By repeating an affirmation many times over days and weeks, you build new neuropathways that encourage you to release unhelpful thought patterns, both conscious and unconscious, supporting a positive shift in mindset.

On the opposite page, I provide a few affirmations for inspiration. I encourage you to write your own, too. Each psyche is unique, and you can best identify the unhelpful thoughts and feelings that you need to reframe. It is likely that these will change throughout pregnancy, so write an affirmation whenever a worry crops up.

The key to writing a powerful affirmation is to make it short, include only positive words, and check that it makes you feel great. Repetition is important, so once you have selected affirmations that will support a positive mindset, introduce them into your life in some of the following ways:

• **Write them on sticky notes** and put them up around your home or workplace
• **Say one in your mind** first thing in the morning, then repeat it regularly throughout the day
• **You and your partner** can say them to each other
• **Listen to** an affirmation audio track
• **When a worry** pops into your head, remind yourself of your affirmation.

"All the strength I need is within me."

"I am calm and relaxed."

"My birth will be positive."

"I relax my mind and my body follows."

"My baby is happy and healthy."

"I take control of what I can and let go of the rest."

"My surges can't be stronger than me; they are me."

"I breathe through every surge."

DEMEDICALIZED TERMS

Words like "contraction" and "pain" settle in your subconscious and guide your feelings about giving birth. Use positive birth-related terms so that birth becomes a joyful, natural life experience in your mind rather than a medical event.

Switch the following medical terms for their more empowering alternatives, and use these going forward. Ask your caregivers to do the same. If they have met hypnobirthing moms, they will be familiar with the following terms already:

- "**Patients**" become "**parents**"
- "**Contractions**" become "**surges**"
- "**Pain**" becomes "**pressure**" or "**sensations**"
- "**Complications**" become "**special circumstances**"
- "**Delivery**" becomes "**birth**"

CHAPTER 1

first trimester

your new pregnancy

A new pregnancy feels truly awesome—it can be delightful and, at the same time, daunting. This exciting time comes with both highs and lows. You might feel amazed at your body's achievement but also apprehensive about how things will turn out.

YOUR CHANGING EMOTIONS

Pregnancy can feel like a strange new land. Even the most yearned-for pregnancy can trigger surprisingly mixed emotions, and many women periodically feel low. With the sharp rise in estrogen and progesterone taking place, your hormones haven't been this wild since puberty. Increased progesterone is associated with the irritability that causes premenstrual tension, and it has the same effect now. Combine this with fatigue, morning sickness, and the uncertainty caused by knowing your life is about to change completely, it's hardly any wonder that pregnant women feel wobbly at times.

Focus on being gentle with yourself during this trimester. Don't judge your feelings—just let them be. You need time to adjust to your changing emotions and new reality. Remind yourself that these hormonal shifts are a necessary part of your pregnancy, enabling your body to nurture the development of your baby and bring her out into the world. Accept your changeable mood in recognition of the vital role these hormones play.

Use the exercises provided in this chapter to help you acknowledge all your feelings and learn to relax deeply. Practice these tools regularly. With a little time, you will learn to foster skills that help you remain serene through any storm.

ACKNOWLEDGE YOUR FATIGUE

During the first trimester, you may feel a profound fatigue, as though you are tired to the depths of your soul. This is because your body is creating another

"

Your mantra can be: all my emotions are valid and welcome.

"

human being! Listen to your body. You may find you don't have the energy to cook or exercise and can barely make it through your workday. Don't feel as though you should power through; instead, slow down and surrender to the feeling. Give yourself as much rest as possible.

MAKE HELPFUL ADJUSTMENTS

There are many small changes you can try to help ease the fatigue and promote deep, restful sleep. Consider the following ideas.

• Rest and retreat whenever possible. Can you take a nap after work? Does the weekend afford more opportunities for catnaps? Even a 15-minute micro-nap can help restore some much-needed energy. Go to bed earlier than usual—

there's no shame in crawling into bed at 8 p.m. or earlier.

• Reduce your social commitments or remove everything from your schedule that is nonessential. You'll catch up with everyone when your energy returns later.

• Ask for help with household chores. This is the time to call in favors from friends and family.

• Disturbed sleep and insomnia often creep in during the first trimester. Try the following: listen to a guided meditation; practice Relaxation Breath (see p.35); take a warm bath with lavender essential oil (see p.45); have a comforting warm drink—camomile tea promotes sleep; take a magnesium supplement (500 mg per day) or have a bath with two cups of magnesium flakes (magnesium chloride) dissolved in it three times a week.

tune in

Learning to tune in to your body and identify your needs is
a valuable skill. It enables you to nurture yourself throughout
pregnancy as your body changes and helps you tap in to
its innate and primal instinct for birthing your baby.

Between work, family, and social commitments, our lives
are often very full. Many women feel pressure to continue
the pace throughout pregnancy and beyond. While this
might be possible, it may not be best for you and your baby.

   This exercise helps you identify what drains or replenishes
your energy. Spend half an hour answering the questions
opposite. Explore each answer in detail, writing notes.
Acknowledge what comes up—it may be unexpected.
Then give yourself permission to prioritize self-care.

   Consider what changes you can make to meet your
current needs. Step back from anything that isn't serving
you. Focus on what makes you happier and more relaxed
rather than what you believe you should be doing.

   Your needs will change throughout the pregnancy, so
repeat this exercise during each trimester and again after
the birth. You may find that the answers change each time.

"

Pamper yourself–luxuries
are now necessities.

"

Which physical or
emotional symptoms are
affecting me?

Which activities or
commitments currently
deplete me?

What brings me
happiness and a sense
of well-being?

your safe space

Your safe space is a visualized inner sanctuary that offers a calm place to retreat to anytime you feel stressed, anxious, or in need of more peace. It can become a helpful tool throughout pregnancy, during the birth itself, and beyond.

Choose a place, real or imaginary, to visualize. It should inspire feelings of joy and peace. Then follow the steps opposite to explore your new sanctuary. Take time to experience emotions fully as you conjure objects, views, people, or animals that make your safe space your ideal haven. Whenever you practice this exercise (do this at least once per week), return to these same elements to enjoy the feelings they inspire. Over time, as you explore your inner sanctuary, adding joyful and inspiring details, the visualization becomes more immersive, and you go into a deeper state of self-hypnosis and relaxation.

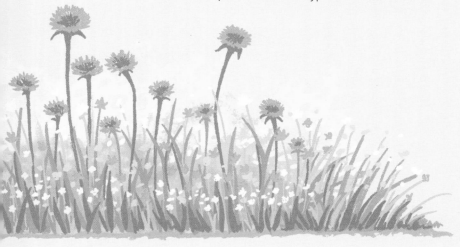

INNER JOURNEY

1

Lie down in a comfortable position. Close your eyes. Slowly breathe in calmness and breathe out tension. Imagine you are in your safe space. What can you see? Conjure anything that makes you feel happy and secure.

2

Focus on smell. What beautiful scents do you smell here? Take a deep breath, as though the sweet smell is filling your entire body.

3

What is the weather like? Is the air warm or cool against your skin? Are there any appealing textures around you to feel? Take a few minutes to enjoy these joyful or soothing details.

4

Notice how your body is reacting to you being in your safe space. Has your heart rate become slow and steady? Take a few deep breaths, release control, and fully surrender to your safe space.

5

Focus on your emotions. How do you feel in your safe space today? Perhaps you feel a sense of belonging, safety, relaxation, peace. Focus on these feelings. Try to increase them.

6

Acknowledge that this feeling of safety is yours. You can tap into it any time by visiting your inner sanctuary. Say goodbye to your safe space and open your eyes.

mutual support

If you are in a relationship, both you and your partner may be experiencing new feelings, some of which may be unexpected or challenging. Use this exercise periodically to explore how each of you feels about your pregnancy and to reconnect.

Teamwork is important in hypnobirthing, and it can begin now with you and your partner cementing a strong, supportive connection with clear, open communication. Use this exercise to help each other navigate the shifting landscape of your lives. Take turns to ask each other the questions opposite. Give the other time to answer each one fully. Be sure you both feel listened to, and work together to put into place changes in response to what you both share. Even small adjustments can have a positive impact. Check in with each other with this exercise regularly.

"

Sharing your worries leads to better connection and teamwork.

"

How are you feeling
this week?

Is there anything you
are worried about?

Is there anything I
can do to help?

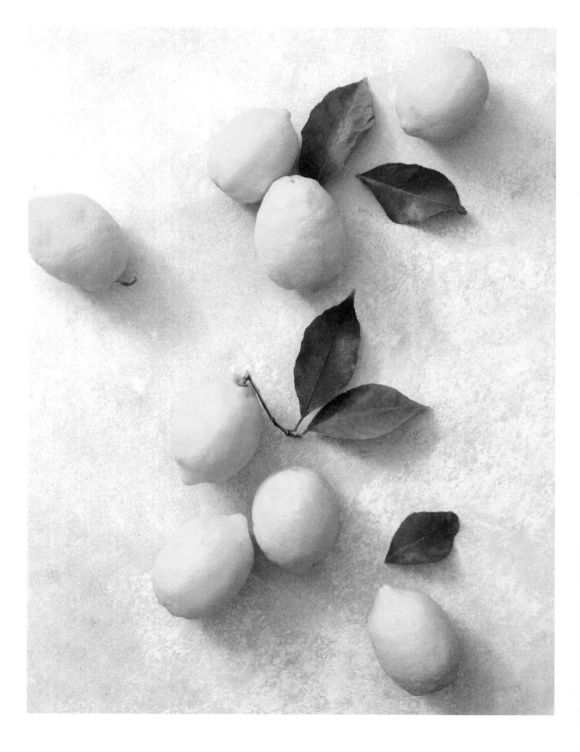

NATURAL REMEDIES

easing morning sickness

Although half of all pregnant women experience morning sickness
during the first trimester, every pregnancy is different, so one person's
tried-and-tested remedy will not necessarily help another. Try
a variety of methods to find those that work for you.

AVOID THE TRIGGERS

It might feel as though anything could set off
your nausea—feeling too hungry or too full,
the smell of food you usually like, or items
like toothpaste or fabric softener. Digestive
complaints (see p.41) can also be triggers.
Avoid your triggers if you can. If necessary,
stick to bland foods like soups, rice, or
mashed potatoes until this phase passes.

EAT LITTLE AND OFTEN

Maintaining stable blood sugar levels by
eating every 1–2 hours (before feeling
hungry) can keep nausea at bay. Try
having six small meals, each including
protein, across the day.

STAY WELL HYDRATED

Keep a bottle of water with you. If you're
struggling with water, try miso or potato
soup or water with fresh lemon, lime,
or mint leaves. Herbal teas are a good
hydration option—ginger, peppermint,
or chamomile teas help relieve nausea.

RELAXATION AND REST

Tiredness can make morning sickness worse.
Opt for early nights and weekend naps.
The deep relaxation experienced using
hypnobirthing tools provides a profoundly
calming distraction from your symptoms.
Try using Relaxation Breath (see p.35) to shift
your focus from your symptoms toward
consciously relaxing both body and mind.

ACUPRESSURE/ACUPUNCTURE

Motion-sickness fabric wristbands can
be worn to stimulate acupressure point
Nei-Kuan or P6. Research indicates that
this effectively reduces nausea and vomiting.
Some women also find that acupuncture
(which is safe during pregnancy) relieves
morning sickness.

ESSENTIAL OILS

Refreshing lemon and uplifting peppermint
essential oils both help ease nausea. Pour 2
drops of your chosen oil onto a tissue, keep it
on you, and take a soothing sniff as needed.

BREATHING TECHNIQUE

relaxation breath

This technique helps you drop down into a state of self-hypnosis and relax deeply. Practice it during pregnancy for a calm journey toward birth, when you can use the tool skillfully to promote a peaceful birth experience.

Relaxation Breath makes you feel calm and grounded, and by reducing adrenaline levels, it helps dispel fear and soothe the nerves. Practice this technique from the first trimester if you can, for a few minutes every day, and at any time you want or need to feel a sense of peace. Lie down on a bed or on the floor, sit in a chair, or sit cross-legged on the floor and follow the steps opposite.

> "
> ## Breathe in calmness and breathe out tension.
> "

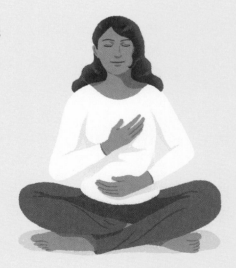

TUNE IN TO THE FLOW

1
Place one hand on your heart and the other on your belly. Close your eyes.

2
Take a long, slow inhalation through your nose and slowly exhale through your nose. Continue to breathe with long, slow inhalations and exhalations.

3
Notice the rise and fall in your chest as you inhale and exhale. Maintain this awareness as you continue to breathe.

4
With each inhalation, imagine drawing in tranquility. With each exhalation, allow tension to release from your face, jaw, and shoulders.

5
Continue to consciously relax with each breath for a few more minutes. Allow any feelings of peace and tranquility to arise as you slowly unwind.

6
Notice how relaxed your body feels. Soak up this feeling and revel in it fully for a few moments before opening your eyes.

PARTNER EXERCISE

guided relaxation

During the birth, your birth partner can be your anchor, helping you feel calm, powerful, and focused on your body. This guided relaxation can be part of their toolkit for supporting you through the early stages.

Practice this 10-minute exercise with your birth partner at least once a week. Sit or lie down comfortably together, holding hands if it reassures you. Your partner asks you to close your eyes and take a few deep breaths, breathing in through your nose and out through your mouth in long, releasing sighs as you relax. Then they explain they will count down from 10 to 1 and, by the time they reach 1, you will feel all tension and stress leave your body. They then read out the guidance opposite, saying the numbers out loud, leaving long gaps between steps. When ready to come out of the relaxation, soak up the feelings for a few moments, then open your eyes.

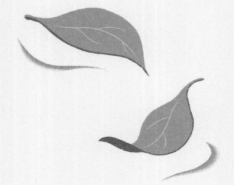

> Your partner or birth partner will find it empowering to be able to guide you into a state of deep relaxation.

COUNTDOWN TO DEEP RELEASE

10

Make any adjustments that will help you feel more comfortable.

9

Become aware of the rhythm of your breath flowing in and out.

8

Relax your shoulders. Allow your chest to expand each time you inhale.

7

Let your jaw soften a little. Allow your tongue and mouth to release.

6

Notice whether any parts of your body remain tense. Allow them to soften.

5

Now begin to let your whole body sink downward into the floor/bed.

4

Allow your body to grow heavier and heavier, sinking further down.

3

Drop down another layer into deeper relaxation.

2

Allow this feeling to grow and flow, grow and flow.

1

You are now feeling deeply peaceful and completely at ease.

MINDSET EXERCISE

fostering self-compassion

We all have an inner critic—the internal voice that's quick to judge
our own thoughts and actions. Pregnancy is a great opportunity
to cultivate your inner advocate—the voice that soothes
the critic and cares for your well-being.

Self-compassion is a useful life skill, and prioritizing
your own needs is an important way of practicing self-
compassion. Over the next few months, reduce your
own expectations of what you can manage. Prioritize
being warm and understanding toward yourself
whenever you feel inadequate. Notice how you speak
to yourself each day. Don't identify with the voice you
hear in your head, but, instead, observe it. Whenever it
is critical, take a few minutes to do this exercise. First,
ask yourself the questions shown opposite. Then use
your answers to help you adjust your inner voice to
nurture and support you in each specific circumstance.
The more you practice this exercise, the stronger the
voice of your inner advocate becomes.

"

Aim for happiness,

not perfection.

"

QUESTIONS

Are you talking to yourself
the way you would to a
sister or best friend?

In this situation, how
would you encourage and
reassure them?

How would you make
them feel safe and loved?

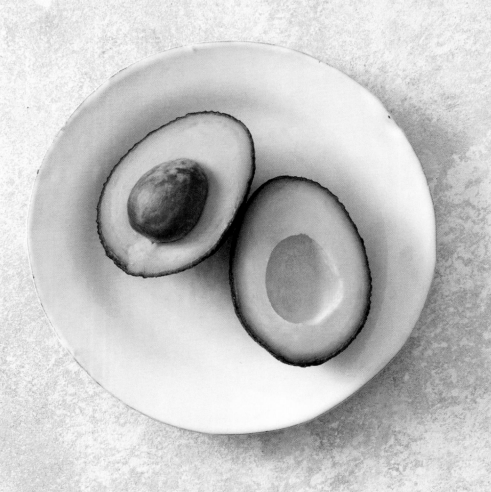

easing digestive symptoms

As levels of the hormone progesterone begin to rise to support your baby's development, digestion slows in response, enabling the gut to absorb more nutrients from the food you eat. This can cause bloating, gas, and constipation. The following remedies may bring some relief.

FOOD CHOICES

If you are surviving morning sickness by eating lots of carbohydrates, this can make constipation worse. Swap refined carbs for protein and vegetables.

Try to sneak some extra fiber into your diet. Snack on popcorn, almonds, pistachios, avocados, vegetable sticks, and fruits. Cut up your favorite fruits to make a fruit salad. Swap white bread and pasta for whole grain versions. Add a side dish of vegetables to your dinner.

If you experience regular constipation, one to three prunes per day or a small glass of prune juice can certainly get things moving.

HYDRATION

Drink a minimum of 68 ounces (2 liters) of fluids daily to keep your stools soft. Use a water bottle to help you keep track of your consumption. Don't forget that herbal teas and soups count as part of your fluid intake.

SUPPLEMENTS

Research shows that regular magnesium supplements can ease constipation. Magnesium citrate is absorbed easily by the body, so choose a pregnancy-friendly brand that your doctor or midwife recommends.

Probiotics (good gut bacteria) may ease your symptoms. Try adding probiotic-rich foods to your diet, such as live yogurt, or take a supplement that contains *Bifidobacterium* or *Lactobacillus* strains.

MOVEMENT

Exercise can stimulate digestion. You may be too tired for your usual exercise routine, so try a regular 15-minute walk or the yoga poses on the following pages.

MINDFUL MOVEMENT

yoga for bloating and gas

The gentle stretches shown here can help bring relief from gas and
bloating. Use them whenever you experience the symptoms. Spend
a few minutes in each pose and notice how your body feels.

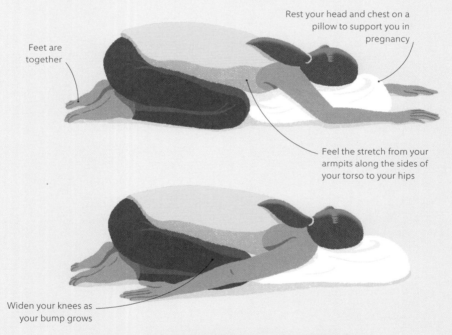

Feet are together

Rest your head and chest on a pillow to support you in pregnancy

Feel the stretch from your armpits along the sides of your torso to your hips

Widen your knees as your bump grows

SUPPORTED CHILD'S POSE

1 Rest on your hands and knees with toes
together and a pillow on the floor below your
head and chest. Sit back on your heels and
lengthen your spine. Exhale, bend forward,
and bring your torso down to your thighs.
Extend your arms forward. Breathe steadily.

2 Bring your arms back to rest alongside
your thighs. Let your arms sink downward,
releasing tension from your shoulders and
neck. Remain in the pose for as long as it
feels good to do so, breathing slowly and
steadily throughout.

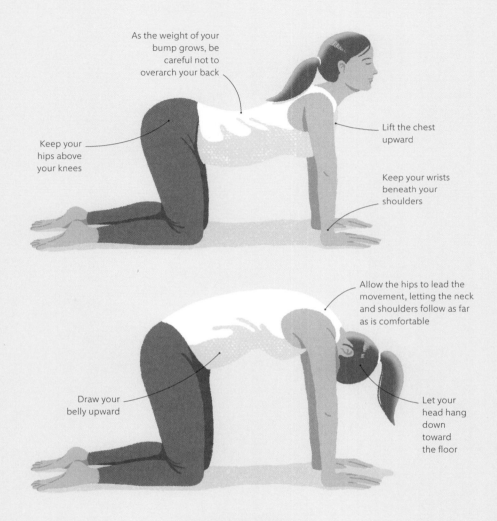

As the weight of your bump grows, be careful not to overarch your back

Lift the chest upward

Keep your hips above your knees

Keep your wrists beneath your shoulders

Allow the hips to lead the movement, letting the neck and shoulders follow as far as is comfortable

Draw your belly upward

Let your head hang down toward the floor

CAT-COW POSE

1 Start on your hands and knees with knees hip-width apart. Move into Cow Pose. Slowly inhale and allow your belly to dip down toward the floor as you lift your chin and chest. Move your shoulders back, away from your ears, and expand your chest.

2 Slowly exhale and move into Cat Pose. Draw your belly (and baby) toward your spine as you release your head down toward the floor. Move slowly between the two postures for a few minutes, ensuring not to overarch your back.

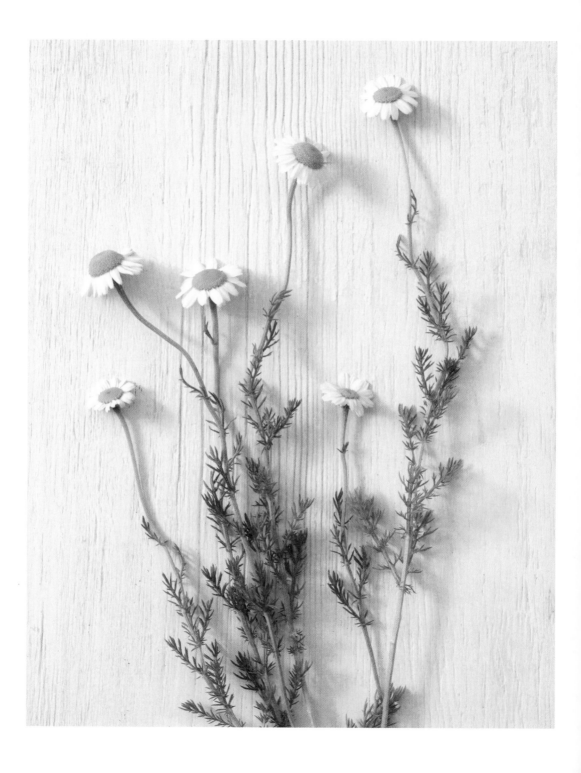

AROMATHERAPY

calm, soothe, and sleep

The soothing properties of essential oils can be harnessed to calm the nerves and relieve aches and pains in the body. This can be a balm during the first trimester, when feeling ravaged by morning sickness and debilitating fatigue.

LAVENDER

Lavender aids relaxation and helps lift the mood. It is also used to promote sleep and soothe aches and pains. Select a product derived from the species *Lavandula angustifolia* (formerly known as *Lavandula officinalis*). This variety is particularly good for soothing aches and pains.

CHAMOMILE

Chamomile soothes the nervous system, promotes a calm state of mind, and improves sleep. It can also be used to reduce morning sickness and stomach upsets. Select the Roman variety of essential oil (known also as *Chamaemelum nobile* and *Anthemis nobilis*).

YLANG-YLANG

Floral ylang-ylang is physically and psychologically calming. It promotes relaxation, soothes the nervous system, and offers a natural aid to sleep. It can help lower blood pressure slightly and boosts the immune system.

HOW TO USE

Place **3 drops** of your chosen oil on your pillow before you go to bed. Lie down and practice Relaxation Breath (see p.35) for a few minutes as you drift off to sleep. See p.156 for further methods of using essential oils.

word of the day

Your focus and intention are potentially powerful forces, and hypnobirthing techniques help you harness them. This daily exercise encourages you to direct your mental energy toward promoting your well-being all day, every day.

Before you get out of bed every morning, use this simple exercise to tune in to your mental, physical, and emotional state and decide how you would like to feel for the rest of the day—then set an intention to focus on promoting that feeling all day long. Keep reminding yourself of your intention throughout the day. This exercise is very useful if you're feeling overwhelmed, since shifting your focus to the positive can help you reframe negative situations.

When you wake up, ask yourself the questions shown opposite to determine where your point of focus should be today. Take a few minutes to consider your answers and select your guiding word. This might be something like "calm," "powerful," "relaxed," "loving," "easy," "fun." Tell yourself three times, "Today will be a calm [*or your chosen word*] day" or "Today I will feel calm," then begin your day.

"

Your focus guides your thoughts and actions.

"

How do I feel today?

How do I want to
feel today?

Which word or
phrase represents
that feeling?

VISUALIZATION

remarkable light

This effective visualization technique appeals to many people, perhaps due to its simplicity. It uses the body-scan method of relaxation to systematically soften your entire body from head to toe, leaving you in a state of serenity and bliss.

Something remarkable is happening in your body. In this exercise, you visualize a light that feels correspondingly special to you that helps you relax. As it sweeps across your skin and penetrates deep within your body, imagine your muscles, organs, and bones softening in response. Reserve 10 minutes once a week for this exercise, and use it whenever you feel overwhelmed or exhausted. With regular practice, you'll be able to give yourself an uplifting emotional boost anytime you need one.

"

Use the light to relax your mind and entire body, inside and out.

"

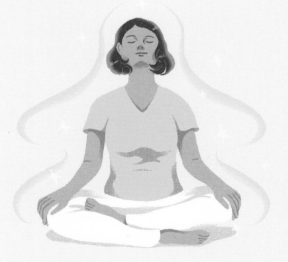

BATHE IN EASE

1

Find a comfortable position, either seated or lying down. Take three slow breaths in through the nose and out through the mouth, allowing your body to grow heavier with each exhalation.

2

Imagine a light shining down on you. It might be sunlight, or you can give it a color or some sparkle. When it shines on part of your body, that area becomes soft and heavy as you release any tension held there.

3

Starting at the crown, the light spreads down to your forehead, across your eyes, upper cheeks, nose, lips, jaw line, and chin, until your entire head is bathed in light and feels soft and relaxed, inside and out.

4

The light shines across your shoulders and shoulder blades, over your chest, across your arms to your fingers. Everything it touches relaxes as the tension lifts away.

5

The light now shines on the sides of your torso, all around your baby, into your lower back and pelvis, over your thighs, knees, calves, ankles, the tops and soles of your feet, and through every toe.

6

Your whole body is now bathed in light and feels soft and relaxed. Soak up this feeling for a minute or two, allowing the light to envelop you. Now slowly open your eyes.

second trimester

boosting your confidence

Your goal is to have a calm and confident mindset for the birth,
so cultivate this state of mind every day. Decide which actions you
can take to promote feelings of peace and tranquility,
and plan them into your daily life.

Every day, practice the skill of creating and returning to a calm and serene internal state. This supports production of the pregnancy hormone oxytocin (see p.11), levels of which are naturally rising in your body.

Continue to prioritize your comfort and peace of mind during this trimester. Don't let rising energy levels tempt you into returning to any punishing prepregnancy schedules. Instead, use the energy to prepare your body and mind for the birth.

FIND YOUR FOCUS

Pregnant women are magnets for all things birth related. Suddenly, everyone wants to share their stories and advice with you. Invaluable nuggets of wisdom are always welcome, but some well-meaning advice can actually increase anxiety and undermine self-belief. It's important to draw away from negativity and look to the positives.

Don't let scary stories worry you. Focus on boosting your own confidence and being calm, by honing the relaxation skills you have been learning. Be mindful about what you engage with—imagine you are wearing a filter that separates stories and information that will support a positive birthing mindset from those that won't. Don't be afraid to stop people if they are scaremongering or

"
Your confidence grows every day with each positive action you take.
"

undermining your confidence. Actively spend more time with those with a supportive outlook or joyful stories to share. Gravitate toward sources of inspiration in books and on social media, and welcome in all the good stuff. Find a yoga teacher that you admire and attend a regular pregnancy yoga class.

CREATE INSPIRATION

Make a visual birth board using images and words that make you feel happy and excited about your own experience. Your pictures could include heavily pregnant women, powerful women birthing, an open flower, blocks of inspiring colors (gold, for instance)—any visual image that you associate with personal power, to remind you to tap in to your own feelings of strength. You could also add birthing affirmations you would like to use in labor. I like the following ones: "Every surge brings me closer to my baby"; "My baby knows what to do"; "I breathe through every surge"; "I look forward to holding my baby in my arms"; "I am powerful"; "I can"; and "I am".

Hang up your birth board in a prominent place so you have a daily reminder of your positive feelings about birthing. It can help you determine your focus throughout the pregnancy and inspire you during the birth itself.

reframe birth

Every woman has a unique perspective on birthing that influences
the feelings that arise when she thinks about giving birth herself.
Exploring your feelings allows you to address any fears you hold
and foster a realistically positive outlook on the process.

Our impressions about giving birth are drawn from stories
we have absorbed from our family, friends, and society.
Use this exercise to examine the inherited stories that
inform you. Give yourself 30 minutes to answer the
questions shown opposite, gently exploring and writing
down your feelings. Take time to read your notes and
reflect on anything unexpected. Acknowledge inherited
fears. Recognize that you can ease them and let them
go (see pp.56–57), that they are negative thoughts and
nothing more—they don't have to be your outcome.
Vision yourself as a powerful woman giving birth and
focus on this image. Write an affirmation (see p.20) to
support your connection to this positive vision, perhaps
"I am strong and powerful" or "My body and I are an
amazing team." Whenever your fears arise, repeat your
affirmation and focus on your vision of birthing power.

"

Tap in to the power and grace women have
used for millennia to birth their babies.

"

What stories about birth
did you hear in your family
while growing up?

What other birth stories
have made an impression
on you?

What is your general
feeling about giving birth?

address your fears

It is helpful for you and your partner or birth partner to take stock of your fears about the birthing process before the event. Practice this exercise together to help you both release any fears you are holding.

Sharing your fears and feeling heard can help you feel lighter and more supported. This exercise is designed to help you deal with your fears as a team. Sit down together for an hour with a pen and paper. Begin by asking one another to locate your level of fear on a scale from 1 to 10 (1 being totally relaxed, 10 being terrified). Note down your chosen numbers. Bear in mind that whatever the number is today, this can be nudged down over the coming weeks as you prepare for the birth and your confidence grows. Now discuss your fears and, for each worry that arises, complete the steps on the opposite page.

> "
> Relax, unfurl,
> and express
> yourselves openly.
> 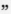"

ACKNOWLEDGE AND AFFIRM

1

Acknowledge your fear by writing it down. Be as specific as possible, which will help you figure out how best to address it.

2

Consider whether you can take any practical actions during pregnancy or the birth to help reduce this concern. Write them down.

3

Write an affirmation in response to this worry. Use positive language to encapsulate how you would rather feel about this particular fear in one sentence.

4

Decide how you will use the affirmation together (see p.20 for guidance).

PARTNER EXERCISE

release fears

Once you have identified your fears (see p.56), use this
visualization exercise to release them symbolically. Regular
practice can help get you into a positive mindset
for birth and boost your confidence.

Spend 10 minutes on this visualization. Ask your birth
partner to read out the steps opposite to help you enter
into a deep state of relaxation. Repeat Step 4 for each
worry you have, imagining you are watching the feeling
of anxiety floating away from you. It is natural to be
apprehensive about the birthing process, especially if
this is your first time. Meeting your birth with confidence,
knowing that you and your baby can do it together,
helps your body relax on the day. So do the work
that will prepare your mind and body for birth (see
pp.102–139) and believe in yourself—you can do this.

LET GO AND RELAX

1

Inhale slowly, then exhale completely, releasing tension from your shoulders with each exhalation. Repeat three times.

2

Imagine you are walking leisurely along a beautiful path. As I count you down from 10 to 1, you will feel more relaxed. *[Count down slowly.]*

3

At the end of the path is a peaceful meadow with a great, wise old oak tree in the center. Under it is a comfortable seat waiting for you. Take your seat.

4

Think of a worry you would like to release. Picture it as a bubble in your hands. Let go of the bubble and watch it drift up to land on a fluffy white cloud above you.

5

Gaze out across the meadow and notice how the clouds are drifting away from you, taking your worries with them. As you watch them vanish, you feel light and peaceful.

6

Take your time to enjoy this feeling of peace. When you are ready, breathe in slowly, relax, and open your eyes.

RELAXATION TECHNIQUE

soft face

It's easy to carry tension in the shoulders, neck, jaw, and face without realizing. This exercise helps you release that tension, and indirectly, it helps you relax the pelvic floor, which is connected to the jaw.

If you clench your teeth, you may be able to feel your pelvic floor muscles become rigid. If you relax the facial muscles, you'll feel release in the pelvic floor. Using the exercise on the opposite page, this response can be put to good use to prepare your body to relax and open during birth. Practice this 5-minute relaxation technique once per week or whenever you notice tension in your face, jaw, neck, or shoulders. It can also be useful if you grind your teeth at night or if you find it hard to relax and let go or identify tension held in your body.

" When you soften your face, your pelvic floor relaxes, too. "

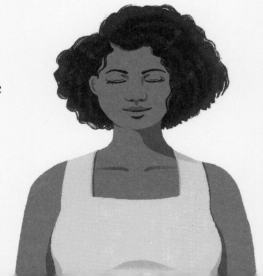

RELEASE AND OPEN

1

Find a comfortable seated position. Pull your shoulders up to your ears, squeeze tight for a couple of seconds, then let them drop down, releasing any tension. Repeat three times.

2

Take a big noisy yawn, stretching out your jaw and mouth. Now close your eyes.

3

Inhale slowly through your nose and exhale through your mouth with a big, releasing sigh. Let your shoulder blades melt down your back with the exhalation. Repeat three times.

4

Allow your jaw to loosen and your lips to part slightly. Allow your tongue to relax in your mouth as you take three slow breaths in and out through your nose.

5

Now focus on your scalp, releasing tension. Now relax your forehead, eyebrows, eyelids, ears, cheeks, nose, lips, teeth, gums, jaw, neck, shoulders, and shoulder blades.

6

Feel the softness in your lower abdomen and pelvic floor. Enjoy the feeling of relaxation for a few moments. Now open your eyes.

BIRTH STORY

"My husband and
I birthed our children
together on our terms,
and our relationship
is stronger than ever
because of it."

Marta, mom to Ernest,
Morris, and Laura

tune in to touch

Soothing touch helps you connect with your body
and mind—and your partner. Asking for the types
of strokes you need fosters trust and
improves communication.

Massage melts away muscle tension and calms the mind. When receiving a massage, your parasympathetic nervous system is activated, which brings many benefits (see p.12). A good massage can reduce stress and anxiety and lead to improved sleep.

Massage also increases levels of the birth hormone oxytocin, so it's a good skill for birth partners to use during the birth. For many women, massage is a cornerstone of their all-important safe and cozy birth environment, providing them with a primal connection to their trusted birth partner.

EXPLORING TOGETHER

If you and your birth partner are new to massage, use these tips to get started:

• Be playful and experiment. If it feels good, then it is good.
• Try massage on the feet, legs, hands and arms, back, and the head.
• Use an appealing oil blend (see p.156).
• Give/ask for feedback as you go—it may take a few tries before you get it just right.
• If you are trying back massage, sit up in a comfortable position—try sitting on a chair backward, with your arms resting on the backrest. Sit topless with a towel wrapped around your front so you feel warm and cozy.
• Your partner should not press down on the spine, which is delicate.
• Allow your mind to quieten as you relax.
• Try to weave in two or three short sessions (15–30 minutes) per week.

CONNECTION EXERCISE

you and your baby

Consciously bonding with your developing baby feels
wonderful, and establishing this bond during pregnancy
can help you focus on your goal during birth—
holding your baby in your arms.

Your body and your little one are working together as an
amazing team, without you having to do anything at all.
Isn't that magical? Use the exercise shown opposite to tap
in to this deeply primal connection. There is no right or
wrong way to do this, so don't worry if you can't visualize
your baby inside. Connecting to the feelings of love and
togetherness is what's important. This exercise takes only
a couple of minutes to perform, so use it any time you
want to feel close to your baby. You can also use it during
birth to give you the strength to power through.

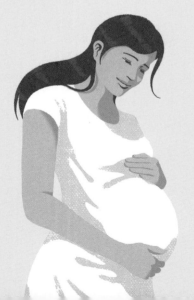

"
You and your
baby are one. She
can feel your love
enveloping her.
"

INTERNAL EMBRACE

1

Sit or lie down in a comfortable position, lay your hands on your belly, and close your eyes. Start to slowly breathe in and out through your nose, feeling your belly rise and fall.

2

Imagine your heart is filling up with love until it feels full to bursting. Give this feeling a color or make it sparkly, if that helps you visualize it.

3

Imagine your love radiating from your heart, moving down your body to flow around your baby abundantly, until she is nestled in the warm, cozy embrace of your love.

4

Now imagine your baby's growing body inside your belly, enveloped in your love. Visualize her little fingers and toes, her arms and legs, and her face smiling back at you.

5

If you have a message for your baby, or would like to say a few words to express your feelings, say them now.

6

Give yourself a minute or two to enjoy this feeling of connection with your baby. Now open your eyes.

BIRTH STORY

"Hypnobirthing wasn't just for me; it was for my partner and for us as a team. It instilled in us a collective confidence in birth by giving him a very specific role and confidence in himself as a supportive birth partner."

Holly, mom to Rufus

your birthing team

Your birthing team includes everyone who will help you prepare for
birth and be with you on the day. If you have a partner, they may
be an obvious choice, and you might consider selecting a
close friend, your sister or mother, or a doula.

Consider carefully who you will ask to join you on this journey. Who will understand your wishes and support you as you need? Many women prefer to have only their partner present during the birth, but having two birth partners can be reassuring for you and for both of them. You may know a second person who would bring something valuable to the team. If your partner is male, having a female birth partner can be reassuring. Lots of good female energy in the birthing room is invaluable.

PREPARE TOGETHER

Your team should prepare for the birth together so that on the big day, you all feel confident and calm. Discuss with them the type of birth experience you want. Don't focus on outcome—instead, explain the atmosphere you want in your birth environment (see pp.114–115), how you would like to feel during the birth (comfortable, safe, tranquil), and what they can do to promote those feelings in you.

Over the next few weeks, encourage your birth partners to feel involved with your pregnancy. Attend appointments and classes together, encourage them to talk, read, and play music to the baby. Practice breathing, relaxation, and massage techniques together regularly. Complete the partner exercises in this book. Write your birth plan together.

CONNECTION EXERCISE

your partner and your baby

If your partner feels connected to the pregnancy, it is easier for them to feel inspired to take positive and supportive actions and remain committed to the hypnobirthing team. Use this exercise to promote a connection between your partner and your baby.

It can be difficult for partners to fully understand that a baby is on the way, because they don't experience any of the physical changes of pregnancy for themselves. Practice this 5-minute exercise regularly to help your partner process the reality of the pregnancy. Sit or lie down together and slowly read out the guidance opposite. Adapt Stage 2 to reflect your changing circumstances. For instance, if your baby is moving, encourage your partner to connect to the active baby in your belly; or if you're aware that your baby's hands and feet will have finished developing, weave in his tiny fingernails and toenails when describing the baby.

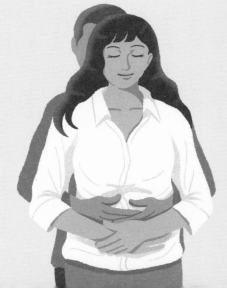

"

Encourage your partner to talk to the baby and touch your belly.

"

VISUALIZE YOUR BABY TOGETHER

1

Place one or both hands on my belly and close your eyes. We will take five slow breaths together, in and out through the nose. As we breathe, be aware of the rise and fall in my belly beneath your hands. Let's begin....

2

As you feel my belly moving, become aware of the amazing life inside. Picture our baby cozy and warm. Perhaps he is sleeping peacefully, or perhaps he is moving inside. Take a little time to connect with your baby right now.

3

Allow in any emotions that this connection brings up for you. All of your feelings are welcome. Take a moment to acknowledge how connecting with your baby makes you feel today.

4

Every day, as our baby grows, he hears your voice and recognizes you. We are all together already. Acknowledge that we are a family. If you have any words you would like to say to the baby or to me, say them now. Open your eyes.

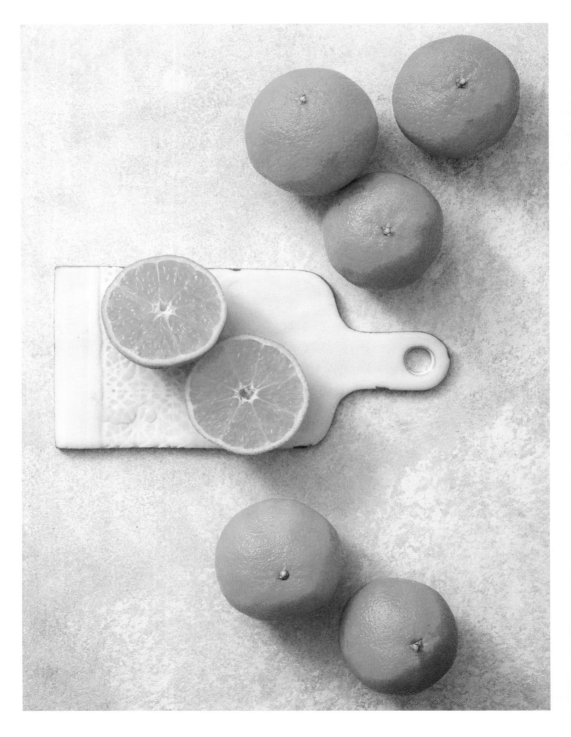

boost your returning energy

Certain essential oils contain antidepressant properties
that can enhance mood. Harnessing these properties
supports the natural rise in energy that women often
experience during the second trimester.

Although fatigue and morning sickness begin to ease, your emotions are likely to remain turbulent at times. Aromatherapy can help increase feelings of balance and ease. The essential oils featured here have mood-enhancing properties, with uplifting and relaxing benefits.

SWEET ORANGE

This uplifting oil harnesses all the magic of citrus. It helps reduce feelings of fatigue and eases anxiety and stress. Sweet orange (see opposite) has antibacterial and mild pain-killing properties, reduces swelling, and stimulates digestion, which helps relieve constipation.

BERGAMOT

The spicy-citrus aroma of bergamot is physically and psychologically calming and can ease muscle aches and digestive upsets. This cleansing essential oil has antiseptic and antibacterial properties and can relieve congested sinuses and ease headaches.

NEROLI

Sweet-floral neroli increases a sense of ease and calm, supporting emotional balance and improved sleep. It has antibacterial and antiviral properties and can relieve constipation, diarrhea, nausea, and cramps—including the twinges of early labor.

HOW TO USE

To support rising energy levels and soothe your nerves, make time for regular relaxation with a soothing weekly aromatherapy bath. See p.156 for directions and other methods of using essential oils.

CHAPTER 3

third trimester

FOCUS ON

slowing down

It may feel as though there are many things to do during the third trimester in preparation for the birth and life beyond it. While that's true, they can all be done at a steady pace as you slow down, ground yourself, and respond to your body's needs.

LISTEN TO YOUR BODY

Throughout this trimester, check in with yourself regularly, assessing how you feel physically. Do you have aches and pains or other symptoms? How connected do you feel with your body? Do you power through when you need to rest? Use these appraisals to decide what will serve you best over the coming weeks.

Now is the time to slow down and prioritize your well-being. Speak to your boss or team if you need to ease the load and tweak your workweek.

Aches and pains are your body's way of talking to you. In Western medicine, we tend to pass off common physical symptoms, like backache, pelvic pain, leg cramps, varicose veins, hemorrhoids, and heartburn, as normal in pregnancy. Traditional systems of medicine, such as Chinese medicine and Ayurveda, work on the principle that all systems in the body are connected, so symptoms can be related rather than looked at and treated in isolation. Common symptoms indicate that the body is out of balance and can be eased by establishing the root cause and treating it with a combination of complementary therapies and conventional medicine, as appropriate.

So if you are having physical symptoms, what is your body is trying to tell you? Try

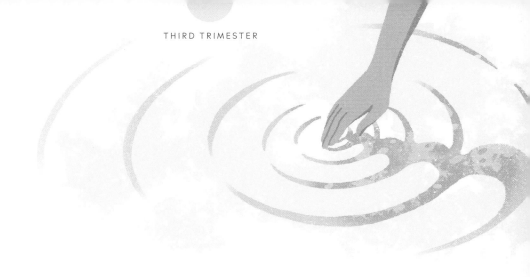

to establish and address the causes of your symptoms in pregnancy, so you don't continue to suffer. Seek the help of an osteopath or physical therapist experienced in working with pregnant women. An acupuncturist may also provide relief. Swimming and yoga (see pp.76–77 and 84–85) can also work wonders for minor aches and pains.

PREPARE FOR THE BIRTH

Taking good care of yourself enables you to build up to the birth in your best condition. In the third trimester, gently prepare your body for birthing while you learn important hypnobirthing tools (see Chapter 4). Practice these skills regularly throughout the third trimester so you are familiar with them on the day.

BUILD YOUR NEST

No doubt you're excited to meet your baby and have him at home with you soon. While you're making plans for how you will meet his needs during the fourth trimester, plan also for meeting your own future needs. Read through the guidance in Chapter 5, which will help you think ahead to the time right after the birth. Use this to make plans and set things in place to help get you on the right track for the rest of motherhood.

MINDFUL MOVEMENT

yoga for strength

Practice this 10-minute sequence daily to strengthen the thighs, bottom, and back in preparation for the birth.

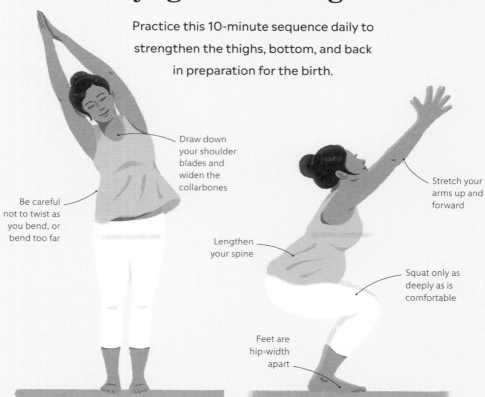

Draw down your shoulder blades and widen the collarbones

Be careful not to twist as you bend, or bend too far

Stretch your arms up and forward

Lengthen your spine

Squat only as deeply as is comfortable

Feet are hip-width apart

SIDE BENDS

1 Inhale and reach your arms over your head. As you exhale, bend to the right from your waist. Take five breaths here. Inhale and return to center, then exhale and repeat on the other side.

CHAIR POSE

2 Exhale, bend your knees, drop your bottom a little way, and raise your arms. Rotate them forward five times, then backward five times, then stand tall.

"
After the sequence, place one hand on your belly and the other on your heart, and send a message of love to your baby.
"

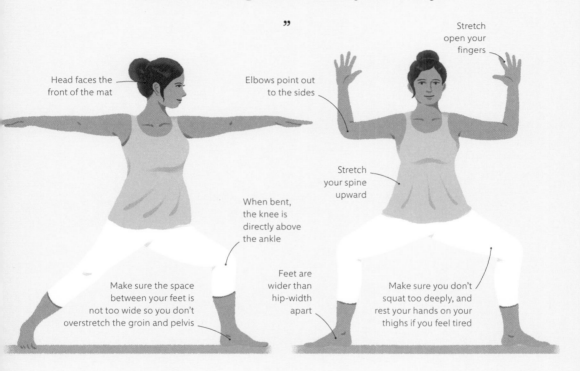

Head faces the front of the mat

Elbows point out to the sides

Stretch open your fingers

Stretch your spine upward

When bent, the knee is directly above the ankle

Make sure the space between your feet is not too wide so you don't overstretch the groin and pelvis

Feet are wider than hip-width apart

Make sure you don't squat too deeply, and rest your hands on your thighs if you feel tired

WARRIOR II POSE

3 Inhale, step your right foot back and bend the left knee. Exhale and raise your arms out to the sides. Hold for as long as is comfortable, then step the right foot to the front of the mat. Repeat on the other side.

GODDESS POSE

4 Turn sideways on your yoga mat. Stand with your feet apart and turn your toes out. Bend the knees and raise your arms with palms facing forward. Take five deep breaths here. Return to the top of the mat.

VISUALIZATION

safe space within

If you have been using the safe space visualization
regularly (see p.29), deepen the practice by inviting
your baby to join you in your inner sanctuary.
Practice this exercise weekly.

If you give birth in a hospital, there may be moments
when your environment doesn't feel comfortable, such
as when traveling to the hospital. By using this visualization,
you will be able to take yourself away into your internal
refuge anytime you need. As before, fully explore your safe
space as you follow the sequence on the opposite page,
anchoring the connection between the things you
visualize and the positive feelings they evoke in you.

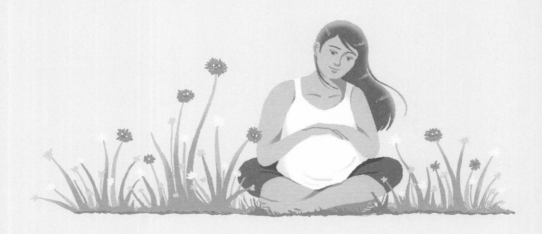

INNER JOURNEY

1

Sit down in a comfortable position, or lay down on your left side. If you are sitting, place a pillow behind your neck and back.

2

Close your eyes and imagine you are in your safe place. Look around you and take in all the meaningful details. Enjoy wandering around, allowing the feelings of comfort, safety, and joy to ebb and flow. Notice how you feel in your body.

3

Now both physically and in your safe space, place your hands on your belly and connect with your baby's presence. Acknowledge that he is with you in your safe space, inside his own safe space within you. You are his home.

4

Invite your baby to share the peace of your safe space with you. Imagine the feeling flowing around you both, and how comfortable and safe your baby feels. Spend a few minutes soaking up these feelings. When ready, slowly open your eyes.

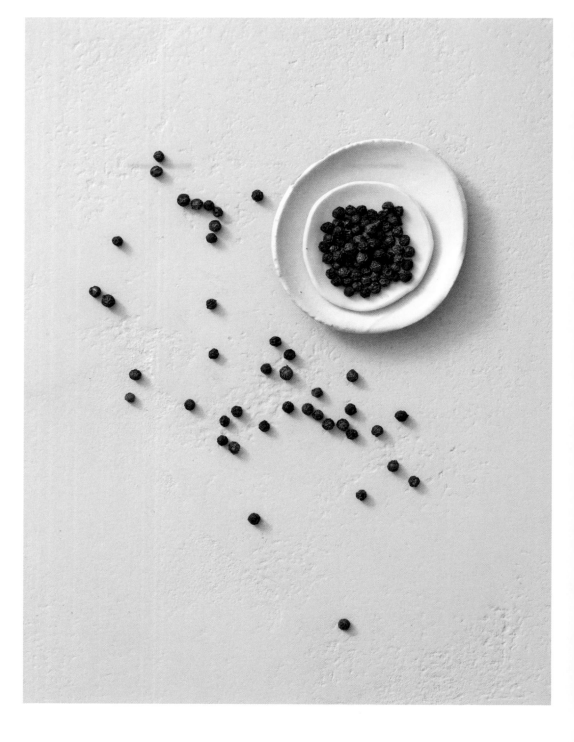

grounding essential oils

As you practice your hypnobirthing tools, aromatherapy can help you quieten your mind and get into the right zone and slow down and connect with your body. These three essential oils are prized for their grounding earth properties.

BLACK PEPPER

Deep, spicy black pepper (see opposite) offers many benefits. It soothes anxiety and can make you feel grounded by helping you feel more comfortable in, and connected to, your body. It soothes gastric symptoms, aids circulation, and brings relief from muscular aches and pains, including backache—which makes it particularly useful at the end of pregnancy and in early labor.

CYPRESS

Herbaceous and woody cypress helps improve circulation and soothe edema (swelling that is caused by a buildup of fluids). This useful essential oil offers antibacterial and antifungal properties, relieves sinus congestion and colds, and aids relaxation.

FRANKINCENSE

The grounding and calming properties of frankincense can help whenever you feel vulnerable. This essential oil relieves general aches and pains as well as congestion, colds, and flu. Choose *Frankincense Carterii* oil.

HOW TO USE

If you plan to use massage during the birth (see pp.122–125), any of these oils can be blended into a comforting massage oil (see p.156) to enrich the experience.

BIRTH STORY

"Hypnobirthing helped me tap into
an internal confidence and know-
how. I learned to respect my body
and mind and trust my intuition.
During pregnancy, I trained for labor:
both in my head, through meditation
and breathing, and in my body,
through physical stretching
and strength building in yoga."

Nicola, mom to Ottilie and Edwin

NATURAL REMEDIES

relieving backache

Backache is common in pregnancy, especially toward the
end. Don't feel you have to put up with it—this is your body
telling you something isn't quite right. There are things
you can try to ease your symptoms.

CHECK YOUR POSTURE

Start by assessing your posture, both when
standing and sitting, especially if you work
at a desk. Sitting forward, propped up
with cushions behind you, or on a birth
ball can help.

If you are sitting throughout the day, be
sure to take breaks every 30–60 minutes to
walk around and stretch your back.

If the problem persists, see an osteopath
or physiotherapist who has experience
working with pregnant women. They will
gently check you over, looking for internal
imbalances and misalignments that might be
causing your symptoms, and make physical
adjustments within the session. It's likely you
will be given exercises to practice at home to
strengthen the problem areas. Often one or
two sessions can relieve discomfort.

MASSAGE

Massage can relieve stiff, painful muscles.
Ask your partner for aromatherapy massages
(see p.81). With a little regular practice, your
partner will learn how to relieve tension in
your problem areas.

MOVEMENT AND EXERCISE

Keep moving so your muscles remain
toned and stretched. Try pregnancy yoga or
Pilates classes or swimming to stretch and
strengthen your back muscles. The Rebozo
technique on p.93 and the yoga postures
overleaf can bring relief from backache.

yoga for backache

The postures shown here and those on pp.76–77 help bring relief from backache as they all stretch the back muscles. Go slowly and listen to your body's feedback, and focus on the postures that help the most.

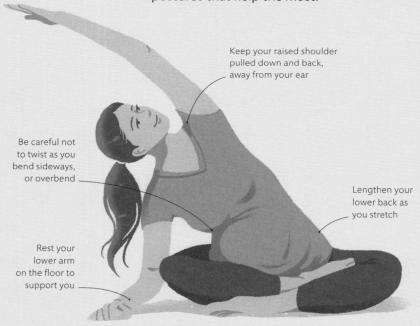

Keep your raised shoulder pulled down and back, away from your ear

Be careful not to twist as you bend sideways, or overbend

Lengthen your lower back as you stretch

Rest your lower arm on the floor to support you

SEATED SIDE BEND

Sit on the floor in a cross-legged position. Inhale slowly through the nose and reach your left arm overhead, allowing the left side of your torso to open. As you exhale, lean over to the right, bending from the waist. Take five slow breaths in this position. Inhale as you return to center, bringing the raised arm to the floor by your side, then exhale. Inhale, reach up with your right arm, then exhale and repeat on the other side.

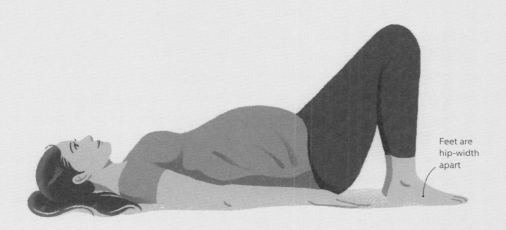

Feet are
hip-width
apart

Knees are hip-width apart—
maintain this distance as you
raise and lower your hips

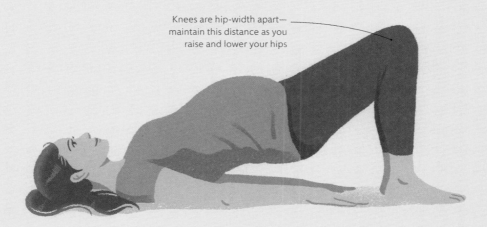

BRIDGE POSE

1 Lie down on your back, then bend your knees and place your feet flat on the floor below your knees. Allow your arms to relax into the floor alongside your body.

2 Inhale, press down into your heels and shoulders, and raise your hips and back off the floor a little. Exhale and lower your hips. Raise and release your hips in sync with your breaths for as long as is comfortable, raising them a little higher each time.

releasing emotional blocks

As you prepare your mind for a positive hypnobirthing experience, it's important not to suppress "bad" emotions. Bottled stress or anxiety can pop up during the birthing process, causing it to slow down or even stop. Use this exercise to help you process challenging emotions.

You're in the third trimester, Mama. Congratulations! How are you feeling? Excited, healthy, calm, tired, uncomfortable? You'll be experiencing a range of feelings, and if you tune in to any difficult emotions, they may point to the areas of your inner landscape in which you have a little work to do. Sit down for 10 minutes and answer the questions opposite in your mind. If anything comes up, whether significant or trivial, try a method of release:
• "Write it out." Spend time journaling, exploring the concern and anything that could help release it.
• Cry! It's okay to cry. Sometimes, this release of tension and emotion is just what we need.
• Talk through the feelings with your partner or a friend. Feeling heard and acknowledged can help us let go of emotions we carry around.

"

All of your feelings, including frustration, anger, and sadness, are welcome.

"

How are you feeling about the birth?

How is your relationship with your partner and your family?

Are you worried about anything at all, no matter how small?

PREPARE YOUR BODY

your baby's position

The position your baby is in when your labor begins
will affect the birthing process. There are lots of things
you can do to encourage your baby into the ideal
position for a comfortable birth.

After 32 weeks of pregnancy, babies tend to settle into one position. If your baby is settling into a position that is potentially more tricky for birth, you can take measures to encourage her to reposition.

At each appointment from 34 weeks, ask your midwife which way your baby is lying and where her back is. If she is not in the ideal anterior position (see opposite, top left), try the following measures.

MIND YOUR POSITION

If you sit leaning backward, you create a hammock at the back of the uterus for your baby to get cozy in. Sit upright, forward, and with legs open (UFO) to encourage your baby to settle at the front. If it helps, prop yourself up with cushions, or sit on a birth ball.

When resting or sleeping, lay on your left side as much as possible. If you need to turn during the night, that is fine, and don't worry if you wake up on your back— just turn back to your left side each time.

If your baby is in a breech or transverse position (see opposite, bottom row), try the inversions shown on p.91.

KEEP ACTIVE

Get moving with walking, swimming, or yoga. After 36 weeks, spend some time every day on your hands and knees or kneeling over a birth ball, chair, or sofa.

Use the Rebozo technique (see p.93) to ease your baby into the anterior position.

SEEK HELP

Consult a pregnancy-specialist osteopath or physical therapist to make sure your pelvis and internal muscles are well aligned. This is particularly important if you are having back or pelvic pain or have damaged your pelvis or lower back in the past.

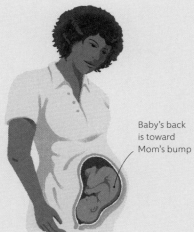

Baby's back
is toward
Mom's bump

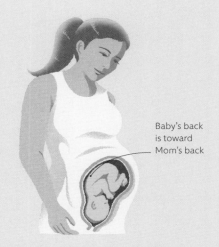

Baby's back
is toward
Mom's back

Occiput anterior In this ideal position, the baby can tuck in her head so it has a small diameter to fit through the pelvis and is lined up to put most pressure on your cervix.

Occiput posterior "Back-to-back" babies often rotate to the front during birth to come through the pelvis. This can slow down the birth, and Mom tends to feel it in her back.

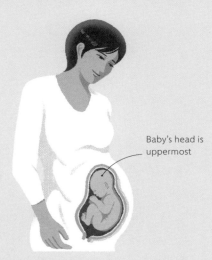

Baby's head is
uppermost

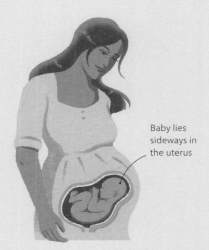

Baby lies
sideways in
the uterus

Breech In some cases of breech, a vaginal birth is still possible, but it is important to find an experienced practitioner. You may be offered ECV (see right).

Transverse Your doctor or midwife may try external cephalic version (ECV) to turn your baby manually from the outside. If she remains transverse, you'll birth by Cesarean.

repositioning your baby

If your baby is in a breech or transverse position, the inverted positions shown opposite can be used from 32 weeks of pregnancy to encourage him to turn to the ideal head-down position (see p.89).

Use these inversions to encourage your baby to turn head down. Practice them, in the sequence shown, two to four times each day for one week. If you feel more kicks at the top of your tummy where the head was and increased pressure in your pelvis, and if your belly has changed shape, it's likely your baby has turned.

Before trying the positions, check with your doctor or midwife that it is safe to do so. Inversions are not suitable for all women. These postures are not recommended if your baby is cephalic (head down), since they can cause him to turn to a breech position. They are also not recommended if you have high blood pressure.

Come out of the positions if you have any abdominal pain or feel dizzy or unwell.

If, after one week, your baby does not turn, see a pregnancy-specialist osteopath or physical therapist to assess and improve pelvic balance, as internal misalignment may be contributing to your baby being in breech position. An acupuncturist may also be able to help.

"
Try to relax if your baby is breech, but be gently proactive about it by doing all you can to encourage him to turn.
"

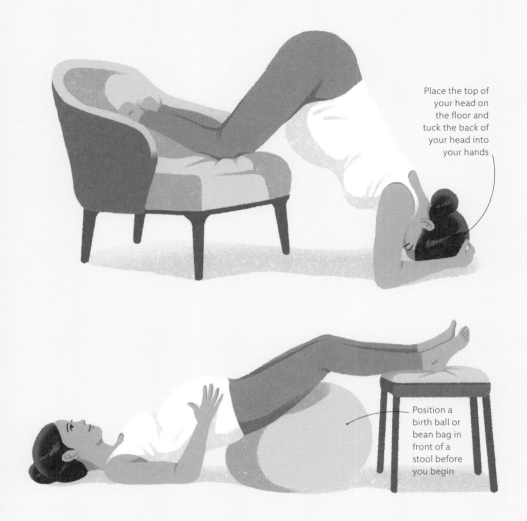

Place the top of your head on the floor and tuck the back of your head into your hands

Position a birth ball or bean bag in front of a stool before you begin

INVERTED POSES FOR TURNING BABY

1 Rest your hands on the floor with your knees and feet on the chair. Carefully lower one forearm at a time to the floor, clasp your hands, and tuck your head into them. Take four slow breaths, then return to kneeling for a pause. Repeat three more times.

2 Lie on your back beside the birth ball. Raise your hips into Bridge pose (see p.85). Slide across so your legs and bottom are well supported and your feet rest on the stool. Stay in position for 10–20 minutes, then ease yourself down onto the floor.

rebozo technique

Indigenous Mexican midwives use a rebozo (traditional
scarf) with this technique to prepare the body for birth
in late pregnancy and to provide relaxation and a
positive distraction during strong labor.

Using a rebozo, the birth partner lifts the belly slightly, bearing the weight of this region during the movement, allowing Mom's muscles and ligaments to relax.

Use this technique in late pregnancy to soothe backache and pelvic pain. If your baby is lying in a posterior position (see p.89), the motion can encourage her to turn to the ideal anterior position.

Practice this technique with your birth partner regularly so that you both feel confident using it during the birth.

Choose a large, fine piece of fabric. During the exercise, you can be on all fours or rest your head and chest on a birth ball or chair. Once you and your partner get into a comfortable swinging motion, find a speed that feels good and continue for up to 5 minutes.

This technique is not recommended if your placenta is anterior (on the front of your belly), if you are expecting twins or multiples, or if you have had any fresh bleeding in the past two weeks.

"

Women find the rocking and jiggling of their body deeply soothing.

"

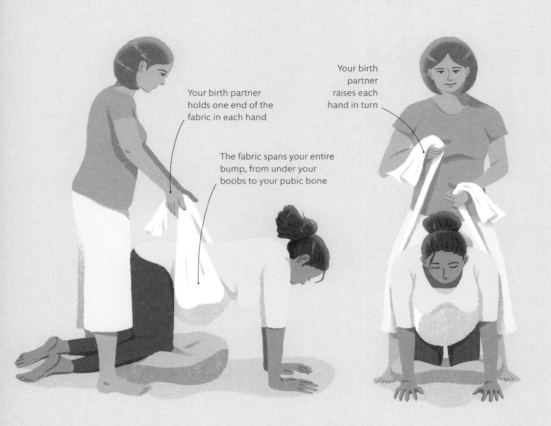

Your birth partner holds one end of the fabric in each hand

Your birth partner raises each hand in turn

The fabric spans your entire bump, from under your boobs to your pubic bone

IN THE SWING

1 Preparation Kneel on a cushion on the floor. Arrange the scarf across your belly to span your entire bump. Your partner stands behind you and takes hold of the scarf at either side of your belly and draws both ends of the fabric toward your back.

2 Swinging motion Your partner slightly raises each hand in turn, gently guiding your hips from side to side, shifting their weight from foot to foot to move in sync with you. To end, they slowly release your belly and help you remove the fabric.

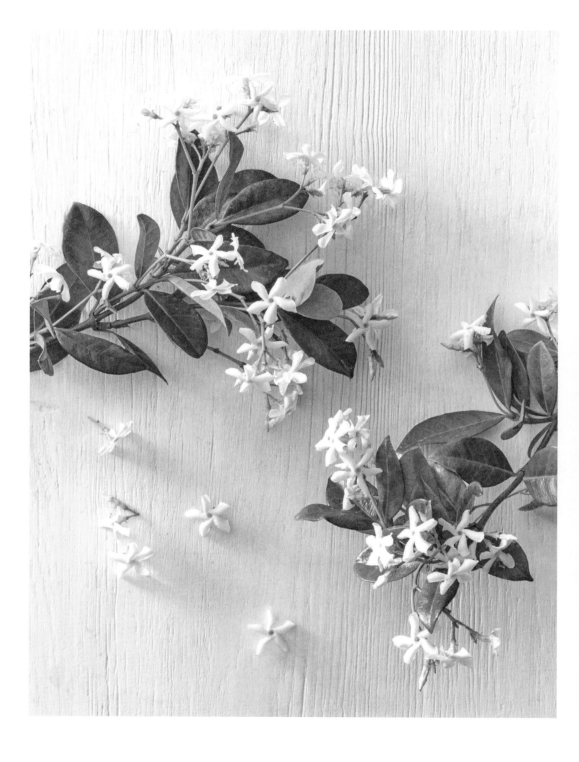

encouraging labor

If offered induction of labor, use any of these soothing, uplifting
essential oils to encourage your labor to begin naturally—but
no more than once per day. Also, use them during labor
to promote strong, long, regular surges.

Caution: Do not use these essential oils prior
to 37 weeks of pregnancy, to avoid activating
labor before your baby has reached full term.

CLARY SAGE

This soothing essential oil has antibacterial
and antiviral properties. During labor, it can
bring on surges, stimulate blood flow to the
womb and pelvis, help reduce blood
pressure, soothe physical sensations, relieve
anxiety, and elevate mood. It can also help
expel a retained placenta after birth.

ROSE

Uplifting rose lifts the mood, calms the
nerves, and stimulates blood flow to the
womb and pelvis. Select *Rosa Damascena* or
Rosa Centifolia oil.

JASMINE

Sweet-smelling jasmine (see opposite) has
antibacterial properties and can bring on
surges, stimulate blood flow to the womb
and pelvis, soothe physical sensations,
relieve anxiety and elevate mood, and help
expel a retained placenta after birth.

HOW TO USE

• **Use a blend** of essential oil and base oil
(see p.156) as a massage oil.

• **Apply 2 drops** of pure essential oil to a tissue
and sniff periodically throughout the day or
during your labor until the aroma wears off.

• **Use in a water** diffuser or, alternatively,
as a spritzer spray (see p.156).

release the pelvic floor

Emphasis is often placed on strengthening the muscles of the pelvic floor, but it is just as important to be able to relax them during birth in order to open, create space, and allow your baby through without causing damage.

The pelvic floor is a "sling" of muscles between your pubic bone and your tailbone that supports the womb, bladder, and bowels. We contract its muscles to stop the flow of urine. Many women have an unconscious habit of keeping the pelvic floor tensed, which is great for keeping the muscles toned but can make it difficult to relax them. Follow this 10-minute exercise to release your pelvic floor muscles. Practice it at least once a week throughout the third trimester. Once comfortable with the exercise, try it in different positions—perhaps on all fours, while sitting, or when in the bath.

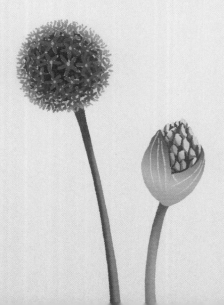

"

Relaxing the pelvic floor eases your baby's way out into the world.

"

RELAX AND OPEN

1

Lie down on a bed or yoga mat with your knees bent and your knees and ankles together. Place both hands on your lower abdomen, below your belly button.

2

Inhale slowly through your nose, then open your mouth and relax your jaw as you slowly exhale through the mouth. Continue for a few breaths, focusing on the rise and fall of your belly.

3

Bring your awareness inside your body, to your pelvic floor. Notice any sensations you feel in this area as you inhale and exhale.

4

Imagine each exhalation traveling down to the pelvic floor to be released, allowing the area to soften more each time. Keep your mouth open and the jaw relaxed. Consciously relax the pelvic floor with each breath for a few minutes.

BIRTH STORY
_____

"Hypnobirthing gave
me confidence in my
own body. It taught me
that birth is not to be
feared and, actually, is
something that my body
is designed to do."

Holly, mom of Rufus

perineal massage

Your perineum is the muscle between your vagina and your bottom. Research suggests that practicing perineal massage for 5 minutes three times per week from 34 weeks of pregnancy reduces the likelihood of experiencing damage to the area during birth.

This massage technique primes the perineum for stretching during birth. It may feel a little strange the first couple of times you try it, but it does become easier. To make it more comfortable, use a gentle massage oil (try almond oil) or lubricant.

HOW TO DO IT

Wash your hands before you begin. Choose a comfortable position in which you can reach your perineum with both hands. You may like to sit at the edge of your bed or stand with one foot on a chair. Smooth some oil or lubricant over the area. Now consciously relax your pelvic floor (see p.97). Position your hands across your groin with your right palm against your right inner thigh and your left palm against your left inner thigh. Place both thumbs inside your vagina as far as the first knuckles. Press your thumbs downward (toward your bottom) to stretch the inside and outside of your vaginal opening and the perineum, using enough pressure to make you feel slightly uncomfortable. Work around the back half of the vaginal opening for 5 minutes. Each time you perform this massage, try to stretch the opening a little more.

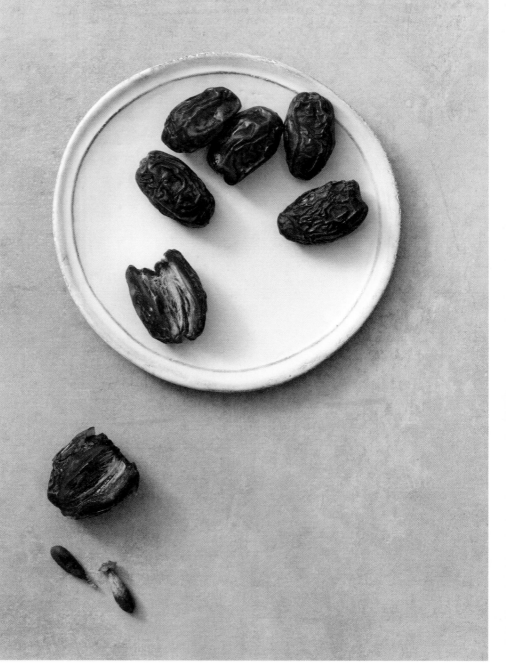

NATURAL REMEDIES

stimulating labor

If you are more than 40 weeks pregnant, or have induction of labor booked, you can take some gentle actions to encourage labor to start naturally. Try any of the following suggestions that appeal to you.

RELAXATION

The hormone oxytocin stimulates labor, and relaxation stimulates its release, so choose activities that support a positive mindset and deep physical relaxation. Use hypnobirthing tools to help you relax. Take self-indulgent time for long baths, yoga, and swimming or to enjoy your hobbies. If you have a partner, have romantic, sensual time together. Also, crying is a good way of releasing tension. Release emotional blocks (see p.86) to help you let go.

MOVEMENT AND TOUCH

Go for vigorous long walks every day, bounce on a birth ball, or do some squats or lunges. All of these activities encourage your pelvis to open and the baby's head to move down.

Nipple stimulation releases oxytocin. One hour of nipple stimulation over a few days can increase your chance of going into spontaneous birth by 30 percent. You can do this with your hands, a breast pump, or your partner's assistance.

ALTERNATIVE THERAPIES

There are several options for stimulating labor. An osteopath can ensure your pelvis is aligned and that your baby is in an optimal position for birth to begin. Reflexology can help you release anxiety and drop down into the hypnobirthing zone. From 37 weeks, an acupuncturist can encourage your cervix to soften and prepare for labor.

EAT DATES

Research suggests that eating six dates per day from 36 weeks of pregnancy reduces the chance of being induced or needing augmentation once birth has begun.

CHAPTER 4

prepare for birth

FOCUS ON

developing your tools

During the third trimester, as you slow down other aspects of your life, turn your attention in a more focused way toward your upcoming birth experience. It's time to learn more about what lies ahead and build up your hypnobirthing tool kit in preparation.

Once you have an understanding of how a woman's body works with her baby during birth (see pp.106–107), you can begin to imagine how the experience might unfold for you and how you could incorporate hypnobirthing tools into the experience to assist you (see pp.108–113).

Thinking this through in advance helps you make appropriate choices for yourself, gather information about your options, and make practical plans for your birth. For instance, you can plan how to set up your birth environment (see pp.114–115) to maximize your chance of a smooth, comfortable birth.

THE HYPNOBIRTHING ZONE

As you make your plans, learn your skills. On pp.118–133, you'll find instructions for a variety of hypnobirthing tools. During the weeks leading up to the birth, practice and hone these skills.

Make a ritual of your practice. As you become more skilled at dropping into a hypnotic state and getting yourself into the hypnobirthing zone, you will boost your confidence about the birth. On the day itself, these skills will become your best friends. Show them to your birth partner, too, who can remind you of them all on the day.

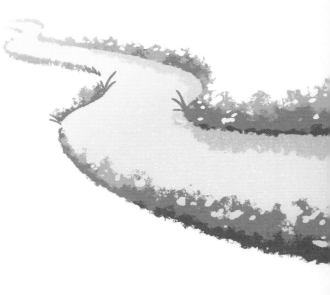

> "
> # Regular practice of your hypnobirthing skills helps you get into the zone.
> "

All this regular practice means you benefit from frequent deep relaxation during pregnancy, bathing your baby in lovely oxytocin. This encourages your birth to start naturally, when the time is right for your body.

PREPARE YOUR BODY

Ease is an important concept in hypnobirthing, and when it comes to your body, you want to ease it toward the birth. During the third trimester, do what you can to get your body into the best physical shape—but do it gently. Build up slowly and maintain strength with yoga postures (see pp.76–77 and 84–85) or some gentle movement, such as swimming and walking.

Encourage your baby into a good position for birth with the deeply relaxing Rebozo technique (see p.93), and practice holding birthing positions you find comfortable (see pp.132–133).

BIRTHING

envisage birth

The body shifts in a miraculous way to allow the baby through the cervix and birth canal. Understanding what is happening helps you feel calm and in control as your body and your baby pass through the different stages of birth.

FIRST STAGE

Medical professionals divide the first stage of labor into two phases: early labor (latent phase) and strong labor (active phase), which ends with the transition to the second stage. During the first stage, the powerful uterine muscle contracts, pushing the baby down and opening the cervix.

Throughout early labor, the cervix softens, shortens, moves up, and opens to 4cm. Surges may feel mild, gaining in regularity and intensity over time.

During strong labor, the cervix dilates to 10cm. Surges become strong, rolling in every 3–4 minutes and lasting for about 60 seconds. Mom can focus on her hypnobirthing tools to ride their intensity. The waters most commonly release during this phase.

Transition occurs when the cervix is 7–10cm dilated and the baby drops down into the pelvis. The cervix and uterus transition from moving up in the body to moving downward, in preparation for the second stage. Surges can come 2–3 minutes apart and last for 90 seconds.

SECOND STAGE

Normally, once the cervix has fully dilated, with each surge the uterine muscles push the baby down through the pelvis and you feel an overwhelming urge to bear down. Once the baby's head emerges, the shoulders emerge one after the other, usually with the next surge, after which the rest of the body is born.

THIRD STAGE

The placenta is expelled during the third stage. If all is well, you can choose to wait for the placenta to come away naturally, which often takes up to an hour, or have an injection of synthetic oxytocin, causing the uterus to contract strongly, which makes the placenta detach from the uterine wall so the midwife can gently pull it out.

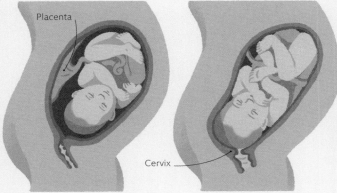

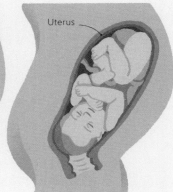

Before the birth begins, your baby is ideally in the anterior position (see p.89). The cervix is firm and closed.

In early labor, the cervix thins and then dilates, opening to 4cm. Here, it is shown at 1cm dilated.

During strong labor, uterine muscles contract frequently to open the cervix further. Here, it is shown at 6cm dilated.

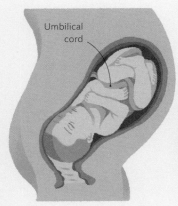
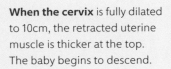

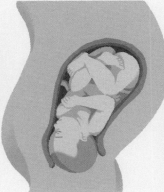

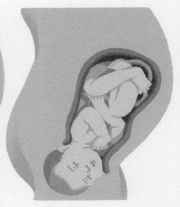

When the cervix is fully dilated to 10cm, the retracted uterine muscle is thicker at the top. The baby begins to descend.

While descending, the baby's head rotates to enable it to navigate the curve in the birth canal and become visible.

The head takes longest to emerge. The body emerges comparatively easily and quickly soon afterward.

BIRTHING

early labor

The rhythm of your birth will be as unique as you and your baby. It may build up gently over a day or two or be powerful from the very first surge. Also, surges feel different for every woman. Be flexible and open minded about your birth so you can meet it as it unfolds.

Until your cervix is 4cm dilated, you are in early labor (see p.106). Relax into this stage and get into the hypnobirthing zone, even if you are induced at the hospital. If at home, distract yourself with your everyday routine. If surges are more than 5 minutes apart or feel light, do things that make you feel happy to boost oxytocin levels. Sleep, lie down and rest quietly, or listen to your hypnobirthing tracks. Practice your Safe Space visualization (see p.79), and start using the Horsey Lips breathing technique to relieve tension (see p.119). Also, try the suggestions opposite. Trust your instincts and do what feels good on the day.

"

Don't rush this first stage—enjoy it. Take your time to enter the hypnobirthing zone.

"

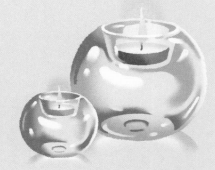

GET INTO THE ZONE

Get physical. Take a walk in nature, do some relaxing yoga stretches (see pp.76–77 and 84–85), bounce on a birth ball, or dance.

Have a relaxing treatment—a pedicure, massage, or reflexology are good options.

Use entertainment to distract yourself. Play board games with your birth partner, do a crossword, or watch a movie or comedy series.

Stroke your pet to release oxytocin, or if you don't have one, watch videos of puppies and kittens on the internet to enjoy their cute factor.

Use a hot-water bottle or wheat bag to soothe your back. The Rebozo technique (see p.93) can help relieve aches, as can the yoga stretches on pp.84–85.

Pamper yourself at home. Have a bath with candles or a refreshing shower. Ask your birth partner for a foot massage using soothing essential oils (see pp.45 and 95).

Eat a delicious meal. Eat now to fuel your body for the birth, as you may not want to eat later on. Perhaps bake a cake, if you enjoy it.

Try using a transcutaneous electrical nerve stimulation (TENS) machine to ease stronger surges. Some women find it offers much pain relief.

BIRTHING

strong labor

When your surges are coming every 3 minutes or so, feel strong, and last for approximately 1 minute each time, the birthing experience becomes more intense. Now is the time to lean heavily on your hypnobirthing tools.

Let your midwife know you've reached this point. It's likely your cervix is anywhere between 4 and 10cm dilated (see p.106). Your tools will help you remain in the hypnobirthing zone throughout this stage. It's helpful to have options to switch between, depending on what you need from moment to moment. The suggestions opposite will be useful. If you've planned a hospital birth, staying at home a little longer, in your own cozy environment, will help. Call the midwife as often as required if you need reassurance, and when you do travel to the hospital, ensure you have planned for a comfortable journey. Continue to use your tools to stay in the zone in transit and once you arrive at the hospital.

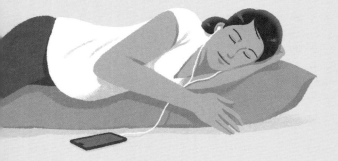

> "
> Each surge is a positive force, bringing you closer to your baby.
> "

STAY ANCHORED IN THE ZONE

Welcome the surges. Use Opening Breath (see p.127) with every surge, or the Dial Down relaxation technique (see p.129) to help reduce their intensity.

Relax between surges. Close your eyes and focus within. Use your Safe Space visualization (see p.79) or listen to a hypnobirthing track.

Keep your mindset steady. Don't worry about how long the process is taking or how dilated your cervix is. Focus on what you can control, be calm, and trust that all is well.

Use aromatherapy. Essential oil on a cool, wet flannel can be soothing. If your surges recede, use an essential oil to stimulate them (see p.95).

Massage can help you feel grounded and safe. See p.123 for massage strokes for this stage.

Laugh! Use the relaxation techniques Horsey Lips (see p.119) and Shaking the Apples (see p.121) to help you laugh, relax, and release tension.

Change position as often as you need. Switch between the active birthing positions shown on p.133. Move around your room and stretch.

A birth pool can offer deep relief. Consider saving it until toward the end of your birth so you have a highly effective tool left to lean on.

BIRTH STORY

"I had found my zone.
My breathing calmed and
I realized I could move and
soften into each contraction.
I thought I could feel my body
opening up, and in a strange
way, I started to find some
bliss in the sensations."

Helen, mom to Ella

BIRTHING

your baby arrives

The transition from the first stage of labor into the second stage
(see p.106) is, for many women, the most intense part of the birthing
process. It helps to remember that you're in the home stretch. Your baby
is moving through your body, out into your waiting arms.

Usually, transition lasts between 30 minutes and 2 hours. During this time, you may feel emotional, overwhelmed, angry, or as though you've hit a wall. This is when women often feel they can't continue and ask for an epidural. Talk this through with your birth partner so they understand it is a normal part of birth. Discuss what they can do to help ease your transition. Massage (see pp.124–125) and lots of reassurance can help. Keep using your hypnobirthing tools. Close your eyes and keep distractions to a minimum.

PUSHING
In many cases, transition leads to a strong urge to push, which guides your baby down and around the curve in your body (see p.107), although some women don't recognize this sensation. Trust your body and follow what you feel. Use Down Breath (see p.131) to keep calm during this stage, which may last around 2 hours with a first baby. Try upright positions (see p.133) or sit on a birth stool or toilet to help your baby navigate through your body.

To help the perineum relax and stretch, ask your midwife to apply a warm compress to the area for a few minutes when the head appears. If possible, the head should be born slowly so the area has time to stretch. Your midwife may guide you by suggesting you blow or pant for the final few pushes. Once your baby is born, he is passed to you. You've done it!

BIRTHING THE PLACENTA NATURALLY
Keep the room cozy and relaxed so the oxytocin is flowing in your bloodstream. To encourage your placenta to emerge, try: breastfeeding your baby or nipple stimulation; using gravity by kneeling up on the bed or standing; emptying your bladder; and sniffing clary sage or jasmine essential oil and rubbing it on your tummy.

your birth environment

What type of space makes you feel relaxed? Which things give you pleasure? Think practically about how to create your ideal hypnobirthing environment, whether birthing in the hospital or at home.

Consider all your senses (see opposite) when planning your birth environment, paying special attention to those that most influence your mood. Find ways of invoking relaxation through your senses, then use these shortcuts to relaxation each time you practice your hypnobirthing tools. They will then keep you anchored in serenity during pregnancy, supporting your hypnobirthing practice, and continue to serve you when you give birth.

"

Birthing hormones flow
abundantly if you are in a place
where you feel safe, loved,
and free of inhibition.

"

DELIGHT YOUR SENSES

Sight Use dimmed lighting to reduce external stimulation and allow yourself to focus on your Safe Space (see p.79). In the dark at nighttime, we release melatonin, which naturally boosts oxytocin, so create a cozy dark ambiance. Try candles, electric candles (in the hospital), fairy lights, using an eye mask or sunglasses, or simply closing your eyes.

Sound Consider which sounds help you relax deeply. This may include your hypnobirthing tracks, your favorite music, nature sounds, or ambient spa music. Silence is an underestimated friend during birth. Many women find music or chitchat irritating. Plan with your birth partner how you will set up your music in the hospital, and prepare a playlist.

Touch You might be soothed by a scented wheat bag, a hot-water bottle, a soft pillow from home, or a cool flannel on your forehead or neck. Human touch can be incredibly soothing. Your partner can hold your hands or give you a massage (see pp.122–125). Some women prefer not to be touched at all during birth.

Smell Use aromatherapy to trigger relaxation whenever you practice your hypnobirthing tools. During birth, use the oils on p.95 to help boost surges. See p.156 for ways in which to use them.

BIRTH STORY

"My birth didn't go to 'plan'–
but I still had the essence of the
birth I wanted. I didn't for one
minute feel robbed of the birth
I had written down. I knew what
was within my control and how to
let go of what wasn't. I knew what
tools I could use however I gave
birth, and I knew that I could still
experience the birth in whichever
way I chose to meet it."

Sophie, mom to Duke and Fela

PLAN AHEAD

your birth plan

Writing a birth plan allows you to think through the event and
consider what tools, techniques, and comforts may work for you.
Make it simple and clear, so your care providers can use it
on the day to help you realize your plans.

Discuss in detail your plans for your birth experience with your birth partner, so they understand what you want and can advocate for you on the day. Together, write your birth plan at 34–36 weeks.

INCOPORATING HYPNOBIRTHING

Include in your birth plan anything that will keep you relaxed and feeling safe, to support oxytocin production. For instance, hypnobirthing moms often ask care providers to use positive language (see p.21). Make a note of how you want your birth environment to feel. Express if you prefer a chattier, encouraging midwife around you or would rather be left in silence to go into the hypnobirthing zone.

PRACTICAL CHOICES

Research your options for birth choices and include them in your birth plan. For example,
consider whether you want vaginal exams; prefer intermittent or continuous monitoring of the baby; do or don't want to be offered pain relief; are choosing active management or the physiological method to birth the placenta; would like the cord to be left intact and, if so, for how long; have requests for helping you maintain the golden hour after birth (see p.145).

PLANS B AND C

It's important to be flexible and acknowledge that, while we can influence much, we can't control everything. Consider various scenarios arising, such as the special circumstances described on pp.136–139. Discuss with your partner how you might manage these. Include your decisions in your birth plan, along with anything that would help you feel calm and in control if things don't go to plan.

BREATHING TECHNIQUE

horsey lips

This technique helps you rapidly release any tension
you are holding in your shoulders, neck, and jaw. Use
it during the birth to relax and ease yourself
into the hypnobirthing zone.

It is useful to find ways of being more present in your body,
so you can consciously relax. Horsey Lips and Shaking the
Apples (see p.121) are techniques that offer easy ways of
doing this, and they may make you giggle and release
oxytocin at the same time. Horsey Lips helps you soften
the jaw and lips, which relaxes the pelvic floor and cervix.
Use it to relieve tension throughout labor, including during
surges. Show your partner the technique so they can
remind you to do it during the birth if you look tense. From
36 weeks of pregnancy, practice it for a minute each day
and whenever you feel tension in your upper back, neck,
or jaw so it becomes an easy, comfortable habit.

"

**It's easy to hold tension
in the body without even
realizing—and just as
easy to release it.**

"

GOOD VIBRATIONS

1

Stand or sit comfortably and with good posture. Now relax your shoulders consciously and allow your shoulder blades to slide down your back.

2

Open your mouth so that your lips are slightly parted, and take a long, slow, deep breath in through your nose.

3

As you exhale through your mouth, shake your head quickly from side to side, release your facial muscles, and allow your lips to vibrate together noisily, like a whinnying horse or a child making a helicopter sound.

4

Repeat the shaking out of your facial muscles for two more breaths. You may not have done this since you were a child, so relax and enjoy yourself!

RELAXATION TECHNIQUE

shaking the apples

This fun, somewhat cheeky relaxation technique relieves tension
in the hips, thighs, and bottom and leaves many in fits of giggles,
increasing that wonderful birthing hormone, oxytocin. It's a
useful technique for a joyful hypnobirthing experience.

Toward the end of pregnancy, many women find that the
weight of their baby pulls on the supporting ligaments,
creating tension in the lower back and buttocks. This may
feel like a dull ache or a sharp, shooting sensation in the
area. When you are tense and stiff, using this technique to
soften up the muscles in this region feels fantastic, and it
helps you bring your attention back into your body.
Practice this technique for 5 minutes twice per week
from 37 weeks of pregnancy, so you and your birth partner
feel comfortable and confident using it during the birth.
It might take a couple of goes before you both get the
hang of it. You will feel everything wiggle internally, and
if that makes you giggle, all the better!

"

Let your birth partner shake
the tension from your hips
while you relax.

"

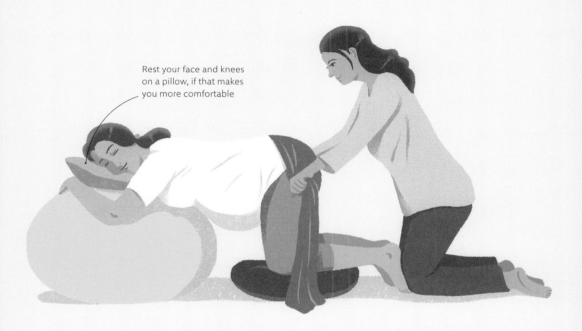

Rest your face and knees on a pillow, if that makes you more comfortable

BE SHAKEN!

1 Kneel comfortably on your hands and knees, or lean on a birth ball or chair. Your partner kneels behind you and arranges the scarf across your buttocks so your entire bottom is snuggled in. They hold one end of the scarf in each hand.

2 Using the scarf to hold your hips, your partner moves them slowly or quickly (as feels good for you) from side to side. Allow your hips to be guided, moving them to your partner's rhythm. Continue for 5 minutes or as long as it feels good.

strokes for labor

Gentle stroking at a speed of 1¼in per second is proven to stimulate pleasure sensations, so ask your partner to use these massage strokes during the birth to help you stay in the hypnobirthing zone.

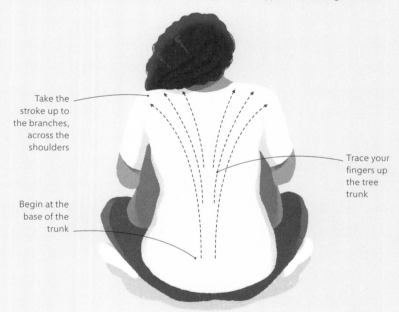

Take the stroke up to the branches, across the shoulders

Trace your fingers up the tree trunk

Begin at the base of the trunk

LIGHT TOUCH TREE

This stroke is great for early labor or if surges have slowed down. Simply trace the shape of a tree on Mom's back. Start at the base of the back, with fingers on either side of the spine, only just touching the skin (use a little more pressure if Mom is ticklish).

Move your fingers slowly upward along the "trunk," then out across the "branches" over the shoulders. Reverse the movements to bring your fingers back to the starting position, then repeat.

"
Soothing touch increases pleasure signals to the brain and boosts levels of birthing hormones.
"

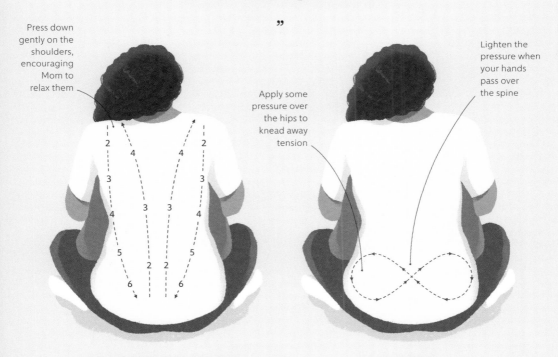

Press down gently on the shoulders, encouraging Mom to relax them

Apply some pressure over the hips to knead away tension

Lighten the pressure when your hands pass over the spine

COUNTING BREATH

During strong labor, guide Mom's breathing in sync with your strokes. Using medium pressure, start at the lower back with a palm on either side of the spine, then stroke upward, saying "Inhale, 2, 3, 4." Press down on the shoulders on 4, then say "Exhale, 2, 3, 4, 5, 6" as you stroke down the sides of the back to the starting position. Repeat.

INFINITY

Place one hand on top of the other in the center of the lower back. Loop around the left hip and come back to center, then loop around the right hip, following the shape of the infinity symbol. Repeat. Move your hands in a smooth, flowing rhythm. This stroke is great for lower-back and hip aches and pains, and in strong labor.

MASSAGE

strokes for transition

When shifting into the transition stage (see p.106), many women feel pressure in their lower back and hips. The massage strokes shown here work particularly well during surges.

Press the palms inward during each surge

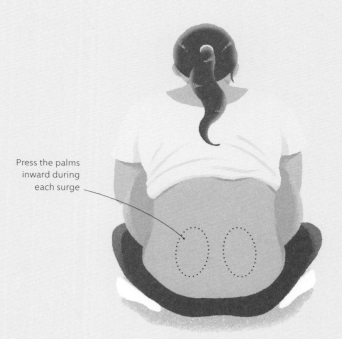

BACK PRESS

Place the hands flat on Mom's lower back, with one palm on either side of her spine, and gently press inward, holding the pressure for around 1 minute or for the duration of the surge. Repeat during each surge. The hands apply heat and pressure to the muscles of the inner back, which can feel amazing for Mom. Be careful not to apply pressure on the spine itself.

"

Allow the heat and pressure from your birth partner's hands to melt away the sensations in your lower back and hips.

"

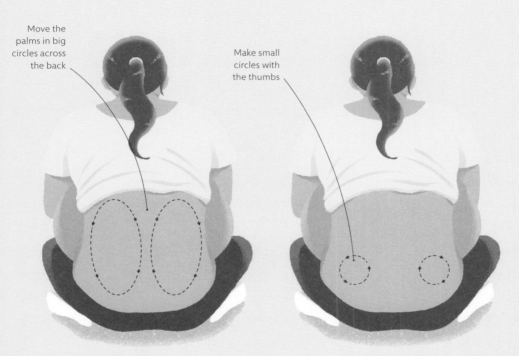

Move the palms in big circles across the back

Make small circles with the thumbs

LARGE CIRCLES

Place the palms on the lower back on either side of the spine. Now draw circles across Mom's back (up and out, down and back in), kneading out tension as you go. Women love this stroke during transition and often ask partners to apply extra pressure.

SMALL CIRCLES

Move the thumbs in small circles on either side of the spine, moving across the region of the lower back and hips. Work the thumbs into any knots or tight spots, applying pressure as guided by Mom. Make sure you do not apply any pressure to the spine itself.

opening breath

This technique helps you relax deeply and drop down into a natural hypnotic state. Use it during birth as your cervix is becoming shorter and opening, perhaps from when you are having one or two surges every 10 minutes.

Start the breath as you feel a surge roll in, and stay with it as the surge rises to a peak and then rolls out. You can stop using the breath when resting between surges. Use this breathing technique to support you during birth until you are fully dilated and feel the urge to push, then switch to Down Breath (see p.131). Practice Opening Breath every day for 5 minutes and twice a week with your partner throughout the third trimester. You can modify the technique to suit you—perhaps inhale and exhale to a set count, or imagine each breath as a wave washing through you. Alternatively, use it as you visualize a soothing scene. Before you begin, find a comfortable position to sit in, place your hands on your belly, close your eyes, and relax your shoulders and jaw.

RIDE THE BREATH

1

Set a comfortable breathing pace as you inhale slowly through the nose and exhale through the mouth.

2

Allow your lips to form a small "O" shape during the exhalation, as though blowing out a candle.

3

Now as you inhale, allow your belly to expand. Pause for a second at the top of the breath, then exhale.

4

Practice for 5 minutes, focusing on the rise and fall of your breath in your belly.

dial down

Every birth is unique, so it is difficult to predict exactly how you will feel while you are having surges. Use the Dial Down hypnobirthing technique to ease your sensations and reduce their intensity.

Grab an ice cube and press it into your palm for 30 seconds. Now observe the sensations. Cold is likely the first thing you notice. But what else is there? Where does your mind go? Does it also feel sharp? Or spicy, or deep? Now repeat the exercise using the Dial Down method on the opposite page. Acknowledge the sensations. As you observe them, consciously "turn them down a notch" in intensity. This will require all your attention. Practice Dial Down in physical postures that fatigue your muscles. Try squatting with your back supported against a wall for 60 seconds. Alternatively, sit with your arms outstretched in front of you, then keep them horizontal to the floor for 2 minutes. Use the steps opposite to reduce the sensations or heat you feel as your muscles work hard.

"

Accept the intensity of the sensation; detach from the feeling.

"

TURN THE DIAL

1

Bring awareness to the part of your body you wish to relax (during birth, this will be wherever you feel your surges—in your belly, back, or both) and pay attention to any sensations you have there.

2

Allow the sensations to just be, and accept them as they are without labeling them as good or bad, pain or pleasure.

3

Imagine that the sensation is reducing, as though you are dialing down a switch on your bodily feelings. Allow the intensity to reduce. Allow yourself to feel more comfortable.

4

See how low you can turn the dial on your perception of the sensations. Can you make it feel as though they have disappeared altogether? When your timed practice ends, take some slow breaths and relax.

BREATHING TECHNIQUE

down breath

When your cervix is fully dilated and the body has started to push involuntarily, Down Breath can help you feel calm and in control, while supporting the body's natural downward focus. It also gets plenty of oxygen in for you and your baby.

Practice this technique from 37 weeks of pregnancy. A great place to practice is on the toilet when pooping! It helps you understand how to use the technique while your body is pushing and releasing downward. Or choose a position in which to practice—try sitting upright, resting on your hands and knees, or kneeling over a birth ball or chair. At the start of this practice, you perform a short exercise (Step 1) to engage the throat. You may feel a slight constriction at the back of your mouth or in the throat. This engagement is what we need to make this breath powerful. Practice Down Breath for 1–2 minutes, then relax. Do not continue a round for any longer, in case you become light-headed.

"

This stage of birth feels primal, so Down Breath can be surprisingly noisy and powerful!

"

RELEASE DOWNWARD

1

Take a deep breath in, then exhale with mouth and throat open, as if steaming up a mirror. Repeat a couple of times with awareness of your throat to engage the area.

2

To begin Down Breath, inhale through the nose, close the mouth (or leave your lips slightly parted), and exhale powerfully down into your throat (air will be coming out of the nose). Continue breathing in this way with slow, deep breaths.

3

Close your eyes. With each exhalation, feel the connection between your throat, diaphragm, and your body all the way down to your pelvic floor. Allow the energy to flow downward. You may notice tightness or heat in your tummy.

4

Now bring in visualization with each breath—imagine the breath is a force like the plunger in a French press, gently moving the baby down through your body. Give this force a color, if it helps you visualize it.

PREPARE THE BODY

positions for birthing

Throughout the birth, it is helpful to change your position regularly to encourage your baby into a good position for navigating the journey through the pelvis. It can help bring relief from aches and pains, too.

Simply changing positions during birth provides relief from discomfort, so shift positions if you are feeling uncomfortable or begin to feel overwhelmed.

Research indicates that using positions in which the body is upright and forward, with hips slightly open (UFO) reduces the length of birth, makes the birth more comfortable and enjoyable for moms, creates space in the pelvis for the baby, and reduces the chance of having an intervention. So avoid lying on the bed throughout the birth.

PRACTICING POSITIONS

There are a number of good positions to use when birthing. Those shown on the opposite page are great contenders. You can also try resting on all fours; Cat/Cow yoga poses (see p.43); kneeling, with your head and chest resting on a birth ball or chair; sitting on a birth ball, resting your head and chest on a bed; sitting on a toilet or birth stool. Try doing Opening Breath (see p.127) in these positions in the last few weeks of pregnancy to see how they feel.

"

Allow your birth partner to help you ease your body from one upright position into another as you birth your baby.

"

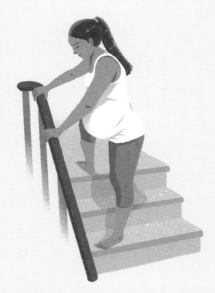

Walk the stairs Walk sideways up and down the stairs, taking them two at a time. This creates space for baby to move down.

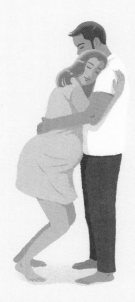

Lean on your birth partner Feel cozy and comfortable, boosting oxytocin, as you lean into the safety of your birth partner.

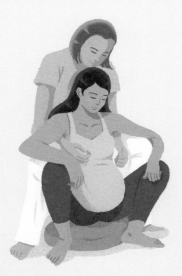

Squat with support This position encourages the baby to make his way down from the pelvis if his head remains high.

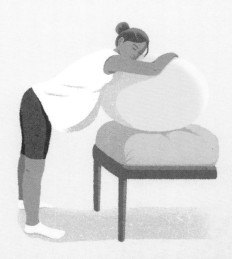

Lean over a birth ball Make the most of gravity while resting in this upright position.

VISUALIZATION

your birth experience

What do hypnobirthing moms have in common with top athletes? Visualization! Visualizing your birth experience, from start to finish, as a normal and healthy birth event will prepare you for exactly that experience.

Brain studies show that visualizing an activity produces the same neurological changes as actually doing it. Research suggests that mental practice is almost as effective as physical practice and can improve your results when it comes to the real deal. This is useful when preparing for birth, as we can't do it for real before the day. Find time to enjoy this visualization regularly from 37 weeks of pregnancy, when you have 10 minutes or more. Good places to practice it are in bed or in the bath, so you can immerse yourself in the feelings of deep relaxation. In your mind's eye, run through the entire event as an uncomplicated birth, from first surge to holding your baby in your arms. Take your time to add vivid details, engaging all your senses.

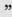

"
How do you want to feel throughout each stage of your birth experience?
"

SEE IT UNFOLD

1

Make yourself comfortable and close your eyes. Take a deep breath in through your nose, and relax your body as you exhale. Repeat twice more.

2

First, picture early labor, with you relaxing at the start then surges slowly becoming more regular. See yourself using Opening Breath (see p.127), remaining calm, and smiling.

3

Your surges intensify. See yourself drop into the hypnobirthing zone. How does the birth room feel? What are you doing? Which birth positions help you relax?

4

Imagine everything inside your body stretching and your cervix opening to fully dilated. You pass through transition and feel your body's strong urge to push your baby down.

5

The baby is moving down with every surge, and you feel powerful and strong. With your body's help, the baby is moving through the birth canal, and he knows just what to do.

6

Picture your baby gently leaving your body, then you holding him cozily against your skin. Lean down to smell his beautiful head and allow the feelings of love to fill your entire body.

BIRTH STORY

"We had a planned induction
and prepared incense, had
relaxing music, dimmed the
lights, and felt excited to
birth. The hypnobirthing
techniques gave us a massive
advantage to feel relaxed and
actually enjoy the process."

Emma, mom to Tilda

planned interventions

It's challenging to be faced with special circumstances (such as a serious medical concern for Mom or the baby) during pregnancy. Use your hypnobirthing tools to help you regain composure and approach the situation from a place of calm and control.

When discussing interventions with your health-care providers, use the **BRAIN** tool to help you remember useful questions to ask:

Benefits What are the benefits?

Risk Are there any risks involved?

Alternatives Are there any? (There often are.)

Instincts How do I feel about it?

Nothing What if we do nothing? The answer to this question can be telling.

Medics make recommendations in line with guidelines based on available evidence, with the average person in mind. These may not cater to your circumstances. Before making choices, look into the research behind the guidelines yourself, and find out whether alternatives are possible.

If you choose a path that is beyond the guidelines, agree to this with your care provider during pregnancy. Ask to meet a consultant midwife or obstetrician to plan this, and go prepared, with written notes, questions, and relevant evidence, and use **BRAIN** to help you stay calm throughout.

POSITIVE CESAREAN BIRTH

If you learn a Cesarean birth is the best option for you and baby, it may take time to release attachment to your original vision of the birth. Let yourself acknowledge and feel this loss.

Take actions toward a positive Cesarean birth experience. Write helpful affirmations, such as "My baby will be born in the right way for him" or "My birth will be calm and magical." Listen to a hypnobirthing track recorded for Cesarean birthing. Visualize your Cesarean birth from start to finish while practicing your Relaxation Breath (see p.35) or Opening Breath (see p.127).

Consider which birth options would make a Cesarean feel empowering and write them into your birth plan. For instance, you may want to take your music into theater; have your birth partner support you with slow breathing throughout; have the screen lowered to see your baby being born; delay baby's first checks so you can enjoy the golden hour undisturbed (see p.145).

managing the unexpected

Things don't always go to plan—but, in most cases, the experience can still be magical. So when you go into birth, be flexible and focus on having a positive birth experience, not a perfect one. Every birthing mother does her best, and, no matter what, you cannot fail at birth.

A long labor can leave Mom very tired and in need of support. In these cases, an oxytocin drip might be used to boost surges, an epidural may be beneficial, or a doctor helps Mom birth with ventouse or forceps. Other common scenarios include when the cervix doesn't fully open or a baby becomes distressed, leading to a Cesarean birth.

MAKING DECISIONS

If you learn that an intervention is suggested, use **BRAIN** (see p. 137) to help you understand what is happening and why so you feel informed and happy with your decisions. Ask for 30 minutes to consider your options before you decide.

Opening Breath (see p.127), Safe Space visualization (see p.79), and your affirmations are your anchors to calm. Use these tools to help you navigate your changing journey. Close your eyes and take yourself into the hypnobirthing zone whenever you need. Once you feel calm, it is much easier to focus on the positives, communicate, and make decisions that feel right.

CONTINUOUS MONITORING

If you are being offered this, ask for the rationale to ensure you need it. You may want to negotiate with the midwife so that you have half an hour of continuous monitoring every 2–4 hours, with intermittent monitoring in between. Ask for a wireless monitor for maximum freedom of movement.

OXYTOCIN DRIP

If you are going to begin or boost labor with an oxytocin drip, try to foster a positive mindset about it. Do what you can to encourage your body to release oxytocin itself. That means relax and boost feelings of love. Focus on how you will soon hold your gorgeous baby in your arms and take him home. Visualize your cervix softening and opening.

BIRTH STORY

"Typically, the birth didn't go to plan! Amazingly, in a time of potential stress, we were both focused and communicated firmly and confidently what we would like to happen next. My partner calmly negotiated with the doctors, and I ended up having a beautiful C-section without any fuss. Thanks to hypnobirthing, we knew what was best at that time, we followed our instincts, and we ended up having a positive experience."

Em, mom to Beau

CHAPTER 5

fourth trimester

your new world

Many foundations are laid during the first three months of your baby's life, so prepare for this important time during pregnancy. Use your hypnobirthing tools to stay positive as you find your way, enabling you to enter motherhood feeling strong and steady.

MEETING YOUR BABY

Your baby is adjusting to her new environment and developing rapidly each day. How you respond to her now makes an enormous difference to how she embraces life. During pregnancy, use the guidance in this chapter to prepare for the fourth trimester so that, when the time arrives, you can focus on your baby and enjoy the experience. She'll pick up on your sense of ease and take it as a cue.

Letting her know she is loved and looked after begins in the precious first hour (see pp.144–145), when you first meet her and get to marvel at her perfection. Allow this process of joyful familiarization to spill into the first week and month.

GIVE YOURSELF TIME

Give yourself a month at home after the birth to strengthen bonds and lay positive foundations. You need time to tune in to your baby and feel your way. This time is quiet and slow, yet you are on constant call, ready to meet the needs of your new baby. Adjusting to the new center of your universe can take weeks, and it's okay to find this challenging.

"

Life with a newborn naturally includes moments of both delight and struggle.

"

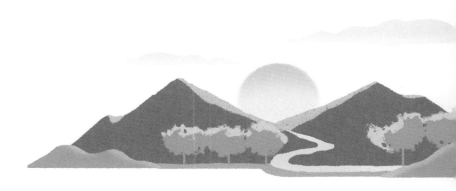

Ease into motherhood (or being Mom to more than one) by figuring out what works for you and your family—not by adhering to what you think motherhood should look like. Release all expectations and focus on being present in each moment. Don't compare yourself to others. Be gentle with yourself and develop trust in your own mothering instincts (see pp.150–151).

HEALING

While your baby is your number-one priority, don't forget that you also have needs. First, you must recover from pregnancy and birth. Rest as much as you can; ensure you eat healing, nurturing foods; and begin your pelvic floor (Kegel) exercises as soon as possible. Many women feel mostly recovered after three months, and it

is normal to need 18 months to feel like yourself again. Rest, recuperate, relax, and enjoy this time with your baby.

USE HYPNOBIRTHING TOOLS

Relaxation exercises can be practiced while breastfeeding and can help breast milk to flow. Opening Breath (see p.127) is excellent if you have sore nipples and helps you stay calm and relaxed while feeding your baby. After birth, the nervous system is often on high alert and sleep is exceptionally light. Use Soft Face (see p.61) or Remarkable Light (see p.49) every day to soothe your body and emotions, and rest whenever you can.

Continue to write and use affirmations (see p.20) to keep your mind clear and your approach focused. Use the exercise Word of the Day (see pp.46–47) whenever you feel overwhelmed.

the first hour

The golden hour after birth is a magical time in which your baby starts adjusting to the world and you begin your lifelong journey together. Take your time to appreciate this pivotal moment that exists between worlds.

If all is well, your baby is snuggled next to you having skin-to-skin contact, which helps regulate his breathing, heart rate, and temperature; reduces stress hormones for you both; and allows you to breastfeed and connect as you try to comprehend how he fit inside your belly. Keep in mind the advice shown opposite as you hold and feed him. If you don't feel well after birth, this golden hour can be shared between your partner and baby and, if disturbed for any reason, recreated later.

> Enjoy the wonder of his
> tiny fingers and toes.

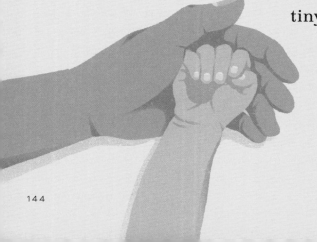

SAVOR THIS SPECIAL MOMENT

1

Be present to delight in the miracle of your newborn. Put away phones—family and friends can wait. Give yourself a few hours cocooned together before visitors come and change the atmosphere.

2

Delay routine checks if you can. Most can be done with your baby on your chest. Those that cannot can wait.

3

Stay cozy. Keep the lights dimmed and the atmosphere calm. If you are in the hospital and are moved after birth, settle in and get comfy in your new space, focusing in on your baby.

4

Relax. After doing such a big job, give your body time to rest. Don't rush to shower and get dressed. Your partner can bring you a toothbrush and a wet face cloth to freshen up if it makes you feel good.

the first week

During the week after birth, stay focused on two things—learning about your baby and healing. Your body has undergone an amazing physical feat and may feel sensitive, bruised, and exhausted.

Spend the first week mostly in bed, wrapped up, eating warming foods, following the guidelines opposite. Don't make plans or do chores. And don't consider this rest a luxury—it is an investment in your long-term health and your family's well-being. Following birth, progesterone and estrogen levels dive, which can make you feel raw emotionally. Try to be present in each moment with your baby. As you get to know her, it will all become easier.

> "
> Now is a time for enormous
> self-compassion.
> "

HEAL IN YOUR COCOON

Use hypnobirthing tools whenever you feel overwhelmed. Try to relax and trust your instincts (see pp.150–151). Use your Safe Space visualization (see p.29) to soothe anxiety and when breastfeeding.

Sleep when your baby sleeps. Accept that she will feed every 1–3 hours and follow her schedule—don't expect her to adjust to yours. Sleep around her needs to fit in lots of healing rest.

Prioritize your physical comfort. Wear soft, baggy cotton clothes and keep warm. Pop a chilled cabbage leaf into your bra to ease sore or engorged breasts. Squeeze breast milk onto cracked nipples to aid healing.

Ask for help. Those closest to you will be pleased to be told what they can do for you. Otherwise, maintain your cocoon and don't feel pressure to have guests over just yet.

PLAN AHEAD

the first month

Plan for the practicalities that will support you during
the first month of your baby's life, enabling you to focus
your energies on forging your bond with him,
as well as on your own self-care.

You'll need help with cooking, cleaning, and perhaps
caring for your other children. You'll also need company
periodically and someone to hold the baby while you
have a nap, shower, or a nurturing treatment. Fill your
freezer with nourishing, warming stews and broths and also
smoothie packs to blend up. Stock up on healthy snacks
such as oat cakes, peanut butter, dark chocolate, dried
fruit, and energy balls. Good nutrition and healthy fats
will balance your hormones, and eating little and often
stabilizes blood sugar levels, reducing anxiety.

"

**Take time to enjoy
the mother-baby
bond you share.**

"

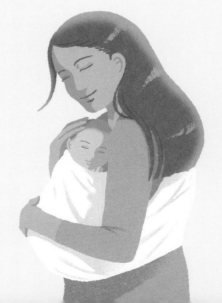

MAINTAIN THE HYPNOBIRTHING ZONE

Ritualize your healing. Use your hypnobirthing practices to keep the happy hormones flowing during this period of transition. Listen to relaxation tracks, have replenishing massages to soothe fatigue, and use aromatherapy (see p.153).

Plan for your comforts. You'll spend hours feeding, so you may want a breastfeeding pillow, a dim side light, a water bottle with a straw, and snacks within easy reach.

Establish a connection with your baby. Stroke his face and talk to him. Sing or read to him. Make eye contact as much as possible. Such connection impacts positively on his neurological and emotional development.

Use a sling to maintain connection with your baby while having hands free to get on with things, or when you go for a walk. Even fussy babies can be soothed in a carrier, and moms find the close connection calming, too.

MINDSET EXERCISE

trust your instincts

Your baby began life as part of you, and you can trust your instincts to nurture her. Use this exercise during the weeks after the birth when, due to sleep deprivation, it can be difficult to make decisions as you adjust to your new world.

During the fourth trimester, you will be getting to know your baby—her habits, her feeding and sleep patterns (or lack thereof!), her noises, what her different cries mean, and how she likes to be held and rocked. So when it comes to her care, trust your intuition, because no one knows her the way you do. It's not always easy to know what you should do. This exercise can help you work through confusion whenever you're faced with a difficult decision or unclear situation. Set aside 10 minutes to ask yourself the questions opposite. Spend a little time really exploring and writing down your answers. When reading them back, consider whether there is any good reason not to follow your instincts. If you find there is conflict between your instinct and what is expected of you, consider how realistic, balanced, or fair that expectation is as part of your decision-making process.

"

Nature has programmed you to know what to do. Go with your gut feelings.

"

What are all my options?

Does my instinct draw me
toward a specific option
or direction?

What do I feel is expected
of me in this situation? And
how do I feel about that?

Setting aside expectations,
what positive actions
can I take, based on
my instincts?

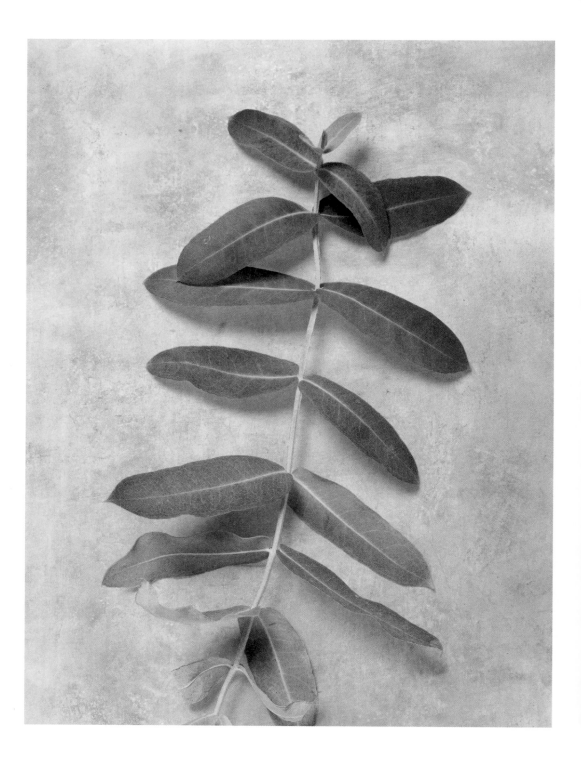

support your healing

Use the essential oils featured below during the weeks after birth
to support your healing and ease emotional or physical tension.
Newborn babies have sensitive skin and a keen sense of smell, so
be careful about how you use essential oils around your baby.

TEA TREE

Tea tree is one of the few essential oils that
you can apply to the skin undiluted. (Add a
few drops to a pad or dressing if applying it
to wounds.) It is wonderful for postpartum
healing, since its antibacterial, antifungal,
antiviral, and anti-microbial properties prevent
wound infection and reduce inflammation.
Use it also as a decongestant for colds and
flu, to relieve anxiety and insomnia, or to
soothe a frazzled nervous system.

EUCALYPTUS

Invigorating eucalyptus (see opposite)
has potent antiviral and antibacterial
properties that help treat cold and flu
symptoms, fever, and body aches. It can
also improve circulation, relieve pain, and
boost the immune system.

MYRRH

Herbaceous and woody myrrh helps balance
emotions, reduce swelling, soothe itchiness,
and promote skin health and healing with its
antibacterial properties. Myrrh can also
support respiratory health and ease asthma,
cough, colds, and lung congestion and can
help relieve indigestion. Note that it is not
safe to use myrrh during pregnancy.

HOW TO USE

- **Sitz bath** Soak a tender and damaged
perineum for 10–20 minutes in a soothing
sitz bath (see p.156).
- **Cool pads** These are chilled sanitary pads
that have been infused with essential oils
(see p.156). Use for postpartum bleeding,
for relief from swelling, stitches, or
hemorrhoids.

maintain the dream team

If you are in a relationship, experiencing the birth together may well have brought you closer. Nourish this connection while navigating early parenthood so that your amazing birthing team becomes a solid, bonded parenting team.

Prioritizing a new baby's many needs changes the existing dynamics in a household, and it takes time to figure out what works for the whole family. Combine this with severe sleep deprivation, feeling raw emotionally, and no time or energy for sex, and you have a recipe for frustration and resentment within your relationship. This exercise helps open the lines of communication, invite in feelings of compassion, increase teamwork, and foster a positive mindset together. Your needs, as well as those of your partner, are likely to change rapidly during this time, so perform this exercise regularly. Give yourselves 20 minutes to ask one another the questions opposite. Acknowledge all the feelings the other expresses, even if you don't agree completely with their answers. Decide on small changes together and set plans in place to implement them.

"

Communicate your needs so you can work together positively.

"

QUESTIONS

Have you enjoyed enough
moments of connection
recently?

Do you feel appreciated for
all the things you do?

Do you need practical help
with anything?

When you need love and
support, is there something
I could say that would help?

using aromatherapy

Throughout this book, I've recommended the use of aromatherapy during pregnancy and birth, suggesting specific essential oils to help alleviate common symptoms.

Aromatherapy is an ancient form of treatment that relies on the aromatic and active compounds in plants to support physical and emotional health. These affect us through the aroma of the essential oil (which, via the brain's sense perception, influences our emotions) and by its absorption through the skin (which has physiological effects).

Traditionally, active compounds are extracted from source plants by cold pressing or distillation. An essential oil is

---

METHODS OF USE

There are a number of ways in which you can use your chosen essential oils, and all of them feel wonderful! Try the methods described here.

If you decide to use more than one oil in a single use, be sure the overall quantity of combined essential oils does not exceed the doses stated.

• **Inhalation**
Put 2 drops of your chosen essential oil onto a tissue, keep it on you, and sniff it periodically until the aroma has diminished.

• **Water diffuser**
Add 5 drops essential oil to the water in your diffuser (normally 3½oz) and allow it to run for 1 hour.

• **Aromatherapy bath**
Run a warm bath. Mix 10 drops essential oil with 1 tablespoon base oil (jojoba, sunflower, coconut, or almond oil). Mix the blend into the bath water.

• **Sitz bath**
Run a warm bath to a depth of 4in. Mix 10 drops essential oil with 1 tablespoon base oil (see left), pour into the bath water, and agitate to distribute the oil. Soak in the sitz bath for 10–20 minutes.

• **Massage**
Add 2 drops essential oil to 1 teaspoon carrier oil (almond, sunflower, or grapeseed oil).

• **Flannel**
Run a flannel under a hot or cold tap, then squeeze out excess water. Add 3 drops essential oil to the flannel and lay it across the back of your neck or on your forehead.

• **Spritzer spray**
Put 20 drops essential oil into a spritzer bottle containing 3½oz water and shake to blend. Use as a facial spray or room freshener. Shake before use.

• **Cool pads**
Mix 2 drops essential oil with 1 tablespoon water. Sprinkle the mixture evenly over a sanitary pad, then pop the pad into a clean bag and refrigerate until cool. Use as a sanitary pad.

therefore a concentrated form of its source material, containing numerous naturally occurring chemicals. Essential oils can be seen as useful and potent "natural drugs" you can use to support your well-being.

To select essential oils for personal use, employ both logic and instinct. If you want something to relieve a physical symptom (such as nausea or muscle aches), make this criteria the basis of your selection. You'll likely find a few essential oils with properties that can soothe your symptom, so to narrow down the selection, choose the one with the aroma that appeals to you most.

There are many ways to enjoy the aromas and benefits of essential oils. Try any of the methods described opposite.

SAFETY

Choose only those essential oils that are safe to use during pregnancy (see right). Whether added to a bath or used in a massage oil blend, essential oils should be diluted before they come into contact with skin. Never apply them directly to the skin since they can cause inflammation or a rash.

Essential oils can make you feel nauseous or give you a headache if overused, so go slowly. If you haven't used them before, start

ESSENTIAL OILS FOR PREGNANCY AND BIRTH

The following essential oils are considered safe to use throughout pregnancy:

- Bergamot
- Black pepper
- Chamomile
- Cypress
- Eucalyptus
- Frankincense
- Geranium
- Lavender

- Lemon
- Neroli
- Peppermint
- Spearmint
- Sweet orange
- Tea tree
- Ylang-ylang

The essential oils listed below are safe to use only after 37 weeks of pregnancy, when your baby is considered to have reached full term, since they can stimulate the onset of labor. This does, however, make them excellent for using during the birth itself, to boost surges:

- Clary sage
- Jasmine

- Rose

by applying your chosen essential oil to a tissue and sniffing it to check whether the selected oil agrees with you or if it causes a reaction. Consult a qualified aromatherapist for further guidance or if in doubt.

INDEX

ABOUT THE AUTHOR

Anthonissa (Nissa) Moger RM is a midwife at St. Thomas' Hospital, London, a hypnobirthing coach, and a yoga instructor who is passionate about improving midwifery practice and birthing conditions worldwide. She believes all women deserve good evidence-based information on pregnancy and birth and, in 2015, established her YouTube channel, The Hypnobirthing Midwife, to make such resources available to a wide audience. In her coaching, Nissa promotes holistic health, combining hypnobirthing with yoga, complementary therapies, and modern midwifery. She runs group sessions in London and virtual classes for international clients and offers free resources on her website (www. thehypnobirthingmidwife.com) that complement the information in this book. Nissa lives with her partner and two children in East London.

ACKNOWLEDGMENTS

From the Author To every single one of my clients, it has been a pleasure and a privilege to support you on your birth journeys, and I continue to be amazed by you! Thank you to Dawn Henderson at DK for giving me the wonderful opportunity to share what I have learned and write this book, and to Salima Hirani for being the best editor I could have hoped for. Finally, a big thank you to my partner, Chris, who supports and champions me in all my endeavors. I love you.
From the Publisher DK thanks Corinne Masciocchi for proofreading, Ruth Ellis for indexing, and Tom Morse for technical support.

DISCLAIMER

Every effort has been made to ensure that the information in this book is complete and accurate. However, neither the publisher nor the author is engaged in rendering professional advice or services to the individual reader. The ideas, advice, and suggestions contained in this book are not intended as a substitute for consulting with your health-care provider. All matters regarding the health of you and your baby require medical supervision. Consult with your health-care provider before undertaking any of the aromatherapy, nutrition, exercises, techniques, natural remedies, and alternative therapies set out in this book. Neither the author nor the publisher shall be liable or responsible for any loss or damage allegedly arising from any information or suggestion in this book.